UNDERSTANDING
DEPRESSION IN WOMEN

UNDERSTANDING
DEPRESSION IN WOMEN

Applying Empirical Research to Practice and Policy

Edited by
Carolyn M. Mazure and
Gwendolyn Puryear Keita

American Psychological Association
Washington, DC

Published by
American Psychological Association
750 First Street, NE
Washington, DC 20002
www.apa.org

To order
APA Order Department
P.O. Box 92984
Washington, DC 20090-2984
Tel: (800) 374-2721
Direct: (202) 336-5510
Fax: (202) 336-5502
TDD/TTY: (202) 336-6123
Online: www.apa.org/books/
E-mail: order@apa.org

In the U.K., Europe, Africa, and the Middle East, copies may be ordered from
American Psychological Association
3 Henrietta Street
Covent Garden, London
WC2E 8LU England

Typeset in Palatino by World Composition Services, Inc., Sterling, VA

Printer: Hamilton Printing, New York, NY
Cover Designer: Aqueous Studio, Bethesda, MD
Technical/Production Editor: Genevieve Gill

The opinions and statements published are the responsibility of the authors, and such opinions and statements do not necessarily represent the policies of the American Psychological Association.

Library of Congress Cataloging-in-Publication Data

Understanding depression in women : applying empirical research to practice and policy / editors Carolyn M. Mazure, Gwendolyn Puryear Keita.— 1st ed.
    p. cm.
Includes bibliographical references and index.
ISBN 1-59147-406-X
1. Depression in women. I. Mazure, Carolyn M. II. Keita, Gwendolyn Puryear.

RC537.U53 2006
616.85′270082—dc22   2005029136

British Library Cataloguing-in-Publication Data
A CIP record is available from the British Library.

Printed in the United States of America
First Edition

Contents

Contributors

Jill M. Cyranowski, PhD, Department of Psychiatry and Psychology, University of Pittsburgh School of Medicine, Pittsburgh, PA

Ellen Frank, PhD, Department of Psychiatry and Psychology, University of Pittsburgh School of Medicine, Pittsburgh, PA

Steven E. Hyman, MD, Provost, Harvard University; Professor of Neurobiology, Harvard Medical School, Cambridge, MA

Gwendolyn Puryear Keita, PhD, Public Interest Directorate, American Psychological Association, Washington, DC

Carolyn M. Mazure, PhD, Department of Psychiatry, Yale University School of Medicine, New Haven, CT

Jeanne Miranda, PhD, UCLA Neuropsychiatric Institute, University of California, Los Angeles

Susan Nolen-Hoeksema, PhD, Department of Psychology, Yale University, New Haven, CT

A. John Rush, MD, University of Texas Southwestern Medical Center at Dallas

Rajita Sinha, PhD, Department of Psychiatry, Yale University School of Medicine, New Haven, CT

Foreword:
The Importance of Studying Women and Depression

Steven E. Hyman

The issue of women and depression is extremely important for public health in general and for the National Institute of Mental Health in particular. Depression is a highly prevalent illness that disproportionately affects women globally. The lifetime prevalence of depression in women is consistently greater than in men in a number of countries and cultures, including the United States, Puerto Rico, New Zealand, France, Iceland, Taiwan, Korea, and Germany (Weissman et al., 1996). Depression is not a cultural artifact, and understanding its pervasiveness and why it affects so many women disproportionately is one of the major goals at the National Institute of Mental Health.

In the past, traditional measures of disease burden, such as prevalence or mortality, underestimated the impact of mental illnesses such as depression. Common colds are widespread but do not have very much economic or health impact. Mortality, when counted at different ages, also has a variable impact. If one dies in one's sleep at age 110, the burden to society is not enormous. A number of years ago, the World Health Organization and the World Bank, in collaboration with the Harvard School of Public Health, developed a better measure of burden called the DALY, or the Disability Adjusted Life Year (Murray & Lopez, 1996). The DALY measures healthy years of life lost, either to premature mortality or to disability. When disability was included as part of the measure of burden, major depression became the second leading cause of disease burden, ranking second only to ischemic heart disease. When disability was examined alone, unipolar major depression was determined to be the leading cause of disability for women worldwide. This discovery came as something of a shock to investigators. When examined more closely, however, these data begin to make a lot of sense. First, depression is highly prevalent. Second, it tends to begin rather early in life and to have a chronic or a recurrent course and, therefore, an enormous impact on disability. It has a disproportionate impact on disability in women not only because of its differential prevalence but also because of the severity of its impact on life course.

As the field of psychology looks toward research, the question is, How is it that gender matters? First, gender provides information about the epidemiology of a disorder. It better characterizes to whom disorders occur and when. Gender also affects the natural history of mental disorders, including mood disorders. For example, depression in some women is related to the stage of their menstrual cycles or to the onset of menopause—obviously gender-related issues. In the case of bipolar disorder, rapid cycling, which can be treatment-refractory and difficult to manage, is far more common in women than in men.

Furthermore, there may be risk factors for mood disorders that differ across gender (Bierut et al., 1999; Nolen-Hoeksema, Larson, & Grayson, 1999). Childhood sexual and physical abuse, which may be very important risk factors for adult depression, disproportionately affect women (Heim et al., 2000; Kendler et al., 2000; Weiss, Longhurst, & Mazure, 1999). This evidence comes largely from retrospective studies but, in aggregate, is quite compelling. Individuals with a history of childhood abuse, either sexual or physical, have an increased risk for depression, and all of the data suggest that women are at much higher risk of being sexually abused as children than are men. Because of problems in reporting and the lack of any standardized criteria for ascertaining abuse or judging its severity, the numbers are not as solid as they could be, but I think that the evidence is convincing. There also is evidence of a dose response relationship. The more severely and chronically a young woman has been abused, the higher the risk of subsequent depression. There have been some interesting studies on the impact of abuse on physiology, partly predicated on some basic science studies in animal models. Women with a history of childhood abuse exhibit increased stress reactivity—that is, activation of their hypothalamic–pituitary–adrenal axis and their autonomic nervous system—in response to laboratory stressors (i.e., public speaking tasks and mental arithmetic tasks with an audience), compared with control subjects who had not been abused. One study showed that for women who have a history of both abuse and major depression, there was a six-fold greater response of the stress hormone adrenocorticotropic hormone than in age-matched control subjects without those conditions (Heim et al., 2000). There is an increasingly solid case for the impact of abuse on physiology and on the risk of major depression.

Some initial work indicates that therapeutics, even pharmacotherapeutics, may differ according to gender. This early evidence indicates that selective serotonin reuptake inhibitors may be more efficacious in premenopausal women, and some of the older tricyclics may actually be more efficacious in men (Kornstein et al., 2000). In addition to pharmacotherapy, gender-specific psychotherapy needs to be examined. Investigation is needed on how to revitalize the area of psychotherapy development with a focus on gender-specific aspects, which might enhance the efficacy of psychotherapy for women.

Gender not only matters in epidemiology, course, risk factors, and therapeutics but also affects people in other ways. For example, there are enormous effects on the families of women experiencing mood disorders such as depression. Maternal depression may act as a risk factor for the onset of depression in a child who also might be vulnerable by reason of shared genes. Sometimes, a central aspect of treating a child with depression is the treatment of other family members who are depressed. At this time, medicine is not always geared toward looking at families but may be excessively focused on the individual child.

Some interesting early evidence, albeit from just a single study in the United States, indicates that depression may have a disproportionate impact on the educational attainments of women compared with men. When men and women have early-onset depression, according to this study, there does not seem to be any difference in their rates of attending college compared with expectation but, disproportionately, women who are afflicted with depression are unlikely to graduate. This lack of a degree, of course, would have an enormous economic impact over the life course (Berndt et al., 2000).

I believe there are salient areas of emerging research, such as the very interesting and important work on risk factors, and areas, such as therapeutics, in which more research is needed on the pathophysiologic reasons why women have twice the occurrence of depression as men. All of this knowledge ultimately must be funneled into improved early recognition for depression and improved treatment that, in light of the disease burden statistics, will have an enormous impact on the quality of lives of women as well as on the lives of families, the health of the nation, and the economy.

References

Berndt, E. R., Koran, L. M., Finkelstein, S. N., Gelenberg, A. J., Kornstein, S. G., Miller, I. M., et al. (2000). Lost human capital from early-onset chronic depression. *American Journal of Psychiatry, 157,* 940–947.

Bierut, L., Heath, A., Bucholz, K., Dinwiddie, S., Madden, P., Statham, D., et al. (1999). Major depressive disorder in a community-based twin sample: Are there different genetic and environmental contributions for men and women? *Archives of General Psychiatry, 56,* 557–563.

Heim, C., Newport, D. J., Heit, S., Graham, Y. P., Wilcox, M., Bonsall, R., et al. (2000, August 2). Pituitary-adrenal and autonomic responses to stress in women after sexual and physical abuse in childhood. *Journal of the American Medical Association, 284,* 592–597.

Kendler, K. S., Bulik, C. M., Silberg, J., Hettema, J. M., Myers, J., & Prescott, C. A. (2000). Childhood sexual abuse and adult psychiatric and substance use disorders in women: An epidemiological and cotwin control analysis. *Archives of General Psychiatry, 57,* 953–959.

Kornstein, S. G., Schatzberg, A. F., Thase, M. E., Yonkers, K. A., McCullough, J. P., Keitner, G. I., et al. (2000). Gender differences in treatment response to sertraline and imipramine in chronic depression. *American Journal of Psychiatry, 157,* 1445–1452.

Murray, C. J., & Lopez, A. D. (Eds.). (1996). *The global burden of disease: A comprehensive assessment of mortality and disability from diseases, injuries, and risk factors in 1990 and projected to 2020.* Boston: Harvard University Press.

Nolen-Hoeksema, S., Larson, J., & Grayson, C. (1999). Explaining the gender difference in depressive symptoms. *Journal of Personality and Social Psychology, 77,* 1061–1072.

Weiss, E. L., Longhurst, J. G., & Mazure, C. M. (1999). Childhood sexual abuse as a risk factor for depression in women: Psychosocial and neurobiological correlates. *American Journal of Psychiatry, 156,* 816–828.

Weissman, M. M., Bland, R. C., Canino, G. J., Faravelli, C., Greenwald, S., Hwu, H. G., et al. (1996, July 24). Cross-national epidemiology of major depression and bipolar disorder. *Journal of the American Medical Association, 276,* 293–299.

Preface

In 1990, the American Psychological Association (APA) published the *Report of the American Psychological Association's National Task Force on Women and Depression* (McGrath, Keita, Strickland, & Russo, 1990), which played a crucial role in highlighting depression as a public health issue, its implications for women, as well as the available treatments.

Since the 1990 Task Force Report, research on depression has increased markedly, expanding our knowledge of risk factors, treatments, and the terrible cost of depression to women, their children and families, and society. The 1990 report made a number of recommendations for methodological advances in research focusing on the health of women, and for specific research targeting enhanced knowledge of risk factors. New research has addressed these issues focusing on women as study participants and on designs that facilitate our understanding of gender differences. From this work, we have especially improved our understanding of the relationship between depression and stress (including different types of victimization), interpersonal styles and relationships, and biological variables (including reproductive events). In addition, the first task force highlighted the need for a greater research emphasis on how the effect of gender may influence treatment considerations. Here, we remain at the early stages of understanding how treatment and prevention initiatives may need to be gender-specific. Yet, we believe initial and continuing efforts in this content area to be essential. The need for improved training of primary care practitioners in screening and treating mental health conditions, as well as building collaboration between general health care providers and mental health professionals, also was highlighted in the earlier report. The data show progress in this area and the value of such training and collaboration; however, sufficient training and close collaboration remain obstacles not yet fully overcome. Finally, the 1990 report recommended research on ethnic minority women, women with co-occurring conditions including substance abuse, and targeted subgroups of women, such as lesbians. As research has increased in these areas, early data support the heterogeneity found in populations of women and the need for further refined examinations of women's mental health.

A decade later, the Summit on Women and Depression 2000 was convened for the purpose of determining which empirical research findings regarding the understanding, detection, treatment, and prevention of depression should be implemented in policy and practice. Researchers and clinicians from multiple disciplines with expertise in depression and related areas provided the most recent information on depression as it relates to women, with the goal of understanding depression from an interdisciplinary perspective and developing recommendations for research efforts in this area over the next 5 to 10 years. *Understanding Depression in Women: Applying Empirical Research to Practice and Policy* is APA's next step in a continued commitment to advancing the field and improving the lives of women.

We are pleased to provide this edited book, divided into four chapters, which addresses the following topics: the etiology of gender differences in depression, treatment and prevention of depression in women, treatment and prevention of depression in targeted populations of women, and effective services for women with depression. We are grateful to the authors of these chapters as well to the experts who attended the APA's Summit on Women and Depression 2000 and contributed essential content (see footnote at the beginning of each chapter). In addition, our thanks are extended to the experts who facilitated discussion for the four substantive areas of the summit: Mary C. Blehar, Lillian Comas-Díaz, Helen L. Coons, Marcy Gross, Miriam Kelty, Vickie M. Mays, Donna E. Stewart, and Susan F. Wood. We are pleased to include a foreword to this volume by Steven E. Hyman who, as the director of the National Institute of Mental Health, participated in opening the summit with a review of research on gender and depression.

We would like to thank Jean Endicott and Marjorie Weishaar for reviewing the manuscript. We especially thank Gabriele Clune, who held the major responsibility for organizing the summit meeting itself, for assisting with the organization of this manuscript, and for editing numerous journal submissions.

We extend our sincere thanks to the agencies and institutes that collaborated with the APA to sponsor the summit. These include the Bureau of Primary Health Care, the U.S. Department of Health and Human Services Office on Women's Health, and the National Institute of Mental Health. Support also was provided by the Agency for Healthcare Research and Quality; the National Heart, Lung, and Blood Institute; the National Institute on Drug Abuse; the National Institute for Occupational Safety and Health; the Office of Behavioral and Social Sciences Research; the U.S. Department of Health and Human Services Office of Research on Women's Health; and the Substance Abuse and Mental Health Services Administration. We also thank the planning committee for the summit and the many individuals who provided guidance and counsel.

Finally, we dedicate this book to all those researchers and practitioners who have sought to understand depression so that the risk of this debilitating disorder is reduced and the suffering caused by depression is abated.

Reference

McGrath, E., Keita, G. P., Strickland, B. R., & Russo, N. F. (1990). *Women and depression: Risk factors and treatment issues.* Washington, DC: American Psychological Association.

UNDERSTANDING
DEPRESSION IN WOMEN

Introduction

Carolyn M. Mazure and Gwendolyn Puryear Keita

The past decade of research has unveiled a great wealth of empirical knowledge on the syndrome of depression. Building on many years of careful inquiry, investigators have begun to explicate the complexity and heterogeneous nature of depression while continuing to confirm that women in the United States and around the world disproportionately experience depression (Weissman et al., 1996). Community-based studies, as early as the 1970s, demonstrated that depression was an especially pressing issue for women. In particular, data generated by the Epidemiological Catchment Area study (Robins & Regier, 1991) provided compelling epidemiological evidence that depression was approximately twice as common in women than in men.

The National Comorbidity Survey (NCS; Kessler, McGonagle, Swartz, Blazer, & Nelson, 1993) replicated and expanded this work, showing that the lifetime prevalence of a major depressive disorder was a staggering 21.3% for women and 12.7% for men. The NCS Replication (NCS–R) data demonstrated overall lifetime prevalence rates of major depression similar to those found in the NCS, and similar relative risk for major depression (Kessler et al., 2003).

Absolute rates of depression for women and men vary by age; however, the gender disparity in lifetime prevalence begins in

3

adolescence and continues into older years. The first onset and subsequent recurrence of depression can occur at any time in life, and depression is the leading cause of disability among women in the world today (Murray & Lopez, 1996). As a consequence, depression is associated with great personal and economic costs (Greenberg, Stiglin, Finkelstein, & Berndt, 1993). The economic burden of depression was estimated at $83.1 billion in 2000, up from $77.4 billion in 1990 (inflation-adjusted dollars). Of these costs, 62% were workplace costs, 31% direct medical costs, and 7% suicide-related mortality costs (Greenberg et al., 2003).

Depression can occur across all educational, socioeconomic, racial, and ethnic groups. Yet, despite the recognition that depression affects diverse populations, the available literature devoted to understanding potential group differences in depressive syndromes is limited. Similarly, depression research examining the interaction of gender across these groups is sparse. Contemporary research increasingly needs to acknowledge the heterogeneity of women and, in this regard, study women from various educational and economic strata and from different racial and ethnic origins.

The four chapters of this volume distill the work of the foremost experts on depression and related fields. As a first step in understanding depression, chapter 1 by Susan Nolen-Hoeksema, "The Etiology of Gender Differences in Depression," explores the causes of and risk factors for depression from psychological, sociocultural, and biological perspectives. It is now known that multiple factors can contribute directly or interact to precipitate the onset of depression. These factors range from environmental stress, including early abusive experience, to cognitive style, hormone and neurotransmitter interactions, and genetics. Stressors implicated in the etiology of depression can be acute or chronic and can incur three times the risk for depression in women than in men. In addition, some precipitating adverse experiences are more prevalent in women than in men, such as childhood sexual abuse, domestic violence, and those experiences generated by lower social status and reduced earning power. Women also appear more likely to develop cognitive perspectives that are associated with increased vulnerability to depression, which in combination with stressors may again enhance the probability of depressive onset. In terms of biological factors that preferentially affect increased rates of depressive onset in women, contemporary data indicate important interactions between neuroregulatory processes and the cyclic effects of gonadal hormones, in addition to genetic factors that may contribute to greater stress reactivity in women than in men. As discussed in chapter 1 (this volume), the new direction of etiological research and the task of new models is to integrate these psychological, social, and biological perspectives as a critical step in understanding the continuing differential prevalence and impact of depression in women.

In chapter 2, "Treatment and Prevention of Depression in Women," Rajita Sinha and A. John Rush provide an overview of the efficacy of psychological and pharmacological interventions, exploring the influence of gender on therapeutic outcome. This overview makes clear that empirically tested treatments are available and should be used. Research clearly shows the success of cognitive–behavioral therapy and interpersonal therapy in treating depression in women, and emerging evidence points to the efficacy of behavioral treatments, including skills training, self-control training, problem-solving therapy, and contingency management.

The efficacy of antidepressant therapy is also highlighted, along with evidence suggesting that women may be preferentially responsive to some antidepressants in contrast to others, and that responsiveness may covary with hormonal status. Current alternative therapies such as acupuncture, herbal agents, and light therapy, though less well studied, also may provide the promise of additional interventions for those who may not be able to or choose not to avail themselves of traditional treatments. An important factor that must be considered in determining treatment strategies is the co-occurrence of depression and other disorders, including substance abuse and personality disorders. These co-occurring conditions can influence depressive outcome and can be treated with specialized interventions.

In chapter 3, "Targeting Populations of Women for Prevention and Treatment of Depression," Jill M. Cyranowski and Ellen Frank show that epochs associated with reproductive life (such as puberty, pregnancy, and perimenopause) deserve a special focus for the development of treatment and prevention strategies, particularly prevention of a first episode of depression. Adolescence presents a unique opportunity for primary prevention of depression by educating preadolescents and their parents, teachers, pediatricians, and others about the risk factors and symptoms of depression, and for interventions to prevent the recurrence of depression. Once a woman reaches childbearing age, she is at heightened risk for depression, with an estimated 9% of pregnant women and 13% of postpartum women experiencing major depressive disorder (MDD). In women with prior episodes of postpartum depression, the risk of postpartum depression in a subsequent pregnancy rises to 25%. With regard to menopausal status, conventional thought has assumed that most women suffer from MDD following menopause. Research has shown this not to be the case but does suggest that women may be at greater risk during the perimenopausal transition. A focus on the epochs in one's reproductive life highlights periods of greatest risk for depression.

In chapter 4, "Improving Services and Outreach for Women With Depression," Jeanne Miranda presents a comprehensive view of the personal, social, and economic costs of depression, as well as the complex relationship between services for depression with race and ethnicity, and socioeconomic status. Women of color and those in poverty have unique needs that require targeted and effective services, yet women of color and those with severely reduced resources have been understudied. The poor and ethnic minorities are particularly vulnerable to receiving limited or inadequate mental health care. Financing of the treatment and prevention of depression in women also is highlighted as a critical issue. Services that are sensitive to women struggling with depression who have children, especially in light of what is being learned about the long-term consequences for these children if their mothers go untreated, is particularly in short supply.

At the end of each chapter are recommendations for the next steps in research and for translating current research findings into practice and into national health care policy. The focus of translation is to use empirically derived data to inform practice.

As defined by the American Psychological Association (APA) Presidential Task Force on Evidence-Based Practice, evidence-based practice is the "integration of the best available research with clinical expertise in the context of patient characteristics, culture, and preferences" (APA, 2005, p. 5). The collaboration of major federal and state agencies with professional organizations in the implementation of these recommendations will enhance access to effective treatment and facilitate the implementation of prevention strategies.

References

American Psychological Association. (2005). *Report of the 2005 Presidential Task Force on Evidence-Based Practice.* Washington, DC: Author.

Greenberg, P. E., Kessler, R. C., Birnbaum, H. G., Leong, S. A., Lowe, S. W., Berglund, P. A., & Corey-Lisle, P. K. (2003). The economic burden of depression in the United States: How did it change between 1990 and 2000? *Journal of Clinical Psychiatry, 64,* 1465–1475.

Greenberg, P. E., Stiglin, L. E., Finkelstein, S. N., & Berndt, E. R. (1993). The economic burden of depression in 1990. *Journal of Clinical Psychology, 54,* 405–418.

Kessler, R. C., McGonagle, K. A., Swartz, M., Blazer, D. G., & Nelson, C. B. (1993). Sex and depression in the National Comorbidity Survey I: Lifetime prevalence, chronicity, and recurrence. *Journal of Affective Disorders, 29,* 85–96.

Kessler, R. C., Berglund, P., Demler, O., Jin, R., Koretz, D., Merikangas, K. R., et al. (2003, June 18). The epidemiology of major depressive disorder: Results from the National Comorbidity Survey Replication. *Journal of the American Medical Association, 289,* 3095–3105.

Murray, C. J., & Lopez, A. D. (1996, November 1). Evidence-based health policy: Lessons from the Global Burden of Disease Study. *Science, 274,* 740–743.

Robins, L. N., & Regier, D. A. (1991). *Psychiatric disorders in America.* New York: Free Press.

Weissman, M. M., Bland, R. C., Canino, G. J., Faravelli, C., Greenwald, S., Hwu, H. G., et al. (1996, July 24). Cross-national epidemiology of major depression and bipolar disorder. *Journal of the American Medical Association, 276,* 293–299.

The Etiology of Gender Differences in Depression

Susan Nolen-Hoeksema

In recent years, three themes have emerged in the literature, providing the basis for contemporary perspectives on gender differences in depression. First, women experience certain stressors more frequently than do men because of women's social roles and status relative to men's roles and sociocultural status, and these stressors contribute to greater rates of depression in

---

Many explanations have been offered for women's greater vulnerability to depression compared with men, and this chapter will provide an integrative review of these explanations. As with other chapters in this volume, this integrative review draws heavily on the contributions of all of the participants of the American Psychological Association's Summit 2000 on Women and Depression but especially focuses on the contributions of the following manuscripts: "Developmental Changes in the Phenomenology of Depression in Girls and Young Women From Childhood Onward" by Maria Kovacs; "Genetic Contributions to the Development of Depression: Are There Gender Differences?" by Laura J. Bierut; "Toward an Animal Model of Female Depression" by Tracy J. Shors; "Psychosocial and Cultural Contributions to Depression in Women" by Vicki S. Helgeson; "Interpersonal Stress and Depression in Women" by Constance Hammen; "Poverty, Inequality, and Discrimination as Sources of Depression Among Women" by Deborah Belle; "Depression, PTSD, and Health Problems in Survivors of Male Violence: Research and Training Initiatives to Facilitate Recovery" by Mary P. Koss; and "Hormones and Mood: From Menarche to Menopause" by Meir Steiner.

women. Second, women may be more prone than men to react to stressors with a depressive outcome as opposed to other forms of psychopathology, because of both biological and socialization-related differences between women and men. Third, more frequent stressors and greater stress reactivity may operate cumulatively to increase rates of depression in women compared with men. Early exposure to adverse childhood events may begin a reciprocal relationship between stress and stress reactivity that perpetuates and kindles women's vulnerability to depression over time. These factors accumulate in the lives of some women and interact with each other to produce depression.

Current Knowledge on the Epidemiology of the Gender Difference in Depression

The gender difference in rates of depression emerges at early adolescence (Kovacs, Obrosky, & Sherrill, 2003; Nolen-Hoeksema & Girgus, 1994). In childhood, boys and girls show similar levels of depressive disorders and depressive symptoms in most studies. When results show a gender difference in prepubertal children, usually boys have greater rates of depression than do girls (Nolen-Hoeksema & Girgus, 1994; Twenge & Nolen-Hoeksema, 2002). Beginning at about age 12, however, girls' rates of depressive symptoms and depressive disorders increase substantially, whereas boys' rates increase only slightly or not at all (e.g., Angold, Costello, & Worthman, 1998; Twenge & Nolen-Hoeksema, 2002). It is also worth noting that boys' rates of substance abuse and criminal behavior increase at this age to a much greater degree than do girls' rates (Angold et al., 1998). By about age 18, the consistent ratio found for females with depression to males with depression in this country is 2:1, and this ratio remains relatively constant throughout the adult life span, although the absolute rates of depression vary across adulthood (Nolen-Hoeksema, 1990, 2002).

Several possible reasons for this gender difference in depression include a greater number of first-onset episodes, longer duration of depressive episodes, a greater recurrence of depression in women than in men, or all of these. Data from three large epidemiological studies conducted in the United States indicate that the greater number of first-onset depressive episodes in women than men, not gender differences in the duration or recurrence of depression, is responsible for this gender difference in depression rates (Eaton et al., 1997; Keller & Shapiro, 1981; Kessler, McGonagle, Swartz, Blazer, & Nelson, 1993; although see Lewinsohn, Clarke, Seeley, & Rohde, 1994). Kovacs, Obrosky, and Sherrill (2003) similarly found no gender differences in the duration or recurrence of depressive disorders in children. As a consequence, the existing literature concludes that women have greater rates of first-onset depression than do men, but once they are depressed, women and men have episodes of similar duration and are equally likely to have recurrent depressive episodes.

Gender Differences in Stressors

Stressful life events are clearly associated with an increased risk for depression (Brown & Harris, 1978; Mazure, 1998), and one hypothesis as to why women have higher rates of depression is that women experience more adverse life events. Some studies suggest that women experience more negative life events in general than do men (Bebbington, Tennant, & Hurry, 1991; Brown & Birley, 1968). Other studies find no gender differences in exposure to negative life events when common stressors in adulthood are sampled (Paykel et al., 1969; Perris, 1984; Uhlenhuth & Paykel, 1973) but do find that the risk for depression associated with severe adverse events is greater for women than for men (Maciejewski, Prigerson, & Mazure, 2001). Also, women experience certain kinds of negative life events more than do men (Kessler & McLeod, 1984; Newcomb, Huba, & Bentler, 1981; Turner & Avison, 1989; Wagner & Compas, 1990; Weiss, Longhurst, & Mazure, 1999). Researchers interested in the relationship of negative life events to greater depressive vulnerability in women compared with men have dealt with the range of events reviewed in the literature in two ways. First, they have focused on specific life events that are more common in women's lives than men's lives because of social roles, rather than looking for gender differences on generic lists of life events. Second, they have investigated the hypothesis that women are more likely than men to respond to a given life event with depression, that is, that women are more reactive than are men to stress.

Physical and Sexual Abuse

In cultures around the world, women are at greater risk than men for suffering several kinds of abuse as a result of their lower levels of social power. Koss, Bailey, Yuan, Herrera, and Lichter (2003) summarized the literature on child sexual abuse, rape, and male partner violence and found ample evidence that the rates of each of these types of abuse are much higher for women than for men. Moreover, abuse is a potent risk factor for depression, both shortly after the abuse occurs and throughout the abuse survivor's lifetime (Weiss et al., 1999). For example, the National Women's Study (Saunders, Kilpatrick, Hanson, Resnick, & Walker, 1999) found that women who had been the victims of completed rape in childhood had a lifetime prevalence of depression of 52%, compared with 27% in nonvictimized women. A meta-analysis of 18 studies of depression and intimate violence found that the mean prevalence rate of depression among battered women was 48% (Golding, 1999). Retrospective studies raise concerns about inaccuracies in memory and reporting, but prospective studies of abused women also provide evidence that abuse increases risk for depression (Widom, 1999). Suicidality, a major and lethal feature of depression, shows especially strong links to a history of abuse (Dube et al., 2001; Oddone-Paolucci, Genius, & Violato, 2001). Childhood physical abuse is the strongest predictor of adult depression in all ethnic groups, after controlling for background characteristics that are risk factors for both abuse and depression.

Sexual and physical abuse may be isolated traumatic events, but more often they occur multiple times at different points across the life span from childhood to old age, and at every stage, women are more likely than men to be victimized. It is unfortunate that prior victimization increases risk for repeat victimization over time (Koss, Bailey, Yuan, Herrara, & Lichter, 2003). Adolescent victimization is the strongest predictor of continued victimization.

Chronic Stress

The lower social status of women compared with men also leads to increased exposure to chronic stressors. Belle and Doucet (2003) showed that poverty is the chronic stressor most consistently correlated with depression in women. Women are significantly more likely than men to have incomes below the poverty line, and high levels of depressive symptoms are common among people with low incomes, particularly mothers with young children (e.g., Belle, Longfellow, & Makosky, 1982; Pearlin & Johnson, 1977). Rates of major depression are twice as high in adults living in poverty, including low-income mothers, as in adults not living in poverty (Bassuk, Buckner, Perloff, & Bassuk, 1998; Brown & Moran, 1997; Bruce, Takeuchi, & Leaf, 1991).

Poverty brings with it an increased risk of a number of acute stressors, including exposure to crime and violence, the illness and death of children, and physical or sexual assault (see Belle & Doucet, 2003). One study of low-income mothers found that 83% had a history of physical or sexual assault (Bassuk, Buckner, Perloff, & Bassuk, 1998). Poverty also brings many chronic, uncontrollable, negative life conditions, including inadequate housing, dangerous neighborhoods, and financial uncertainties. The stresses of poverty can undermine parenting skills, increase marital conflict, reduce self-esteem, and limit coping strategies. In addition, poor women may turn to family and friends for support, but they may also be poor, and perceived stress can be increased in the entire social network through social contagion (Belle & Doucet, 2003).

Gender inequalities exist not only in rates of extreme poverty but throughout the economic ladder, with working women making only 74 cents for every dollar working men make (U.S. Census Bureau, 2004). The income gap between women and men has been narrowing in recent years, but this is primarily due to decreases in men's real wages, not to increases in women's wages (U.S. Census Bureau, 2004). In turn, an association between socioeconomic status (SES) and depression exists at all levels of the SES hierarchy. For example, Eaton and Muntaner (1999) found that people whose household income was less than $17,500 were 16 times more likely to be diagnosed with major depressive disorder than were those whose household income was over $35,000, whereas those with household incomes in the middle range were 11 times more likely to be diagnosed with major depressive disorder. Few studies have specifically examined the effects of gender differences in income across all SES levels on the gender difference in depression.

Another chronic stressor in some women's lives is *discrimination*, defined as a process in which the dominant group's privileges are maintained at the expense of a subordinate group (Feagin & Feagin, 1978). Landrine, Klonoff, Gibbs, Maning, and Lund (1995) found that sexist discrimination against women (e.g., being treated unfairly on the job because one is a woman) accounted for more variance in depressive symptoms among women than did standard measures of life events and hassles. Women's reporting of recent and lifetime sex discrimination entirely accounted for the observed differences between women and men in depressive symptoms in a student sample (Klonoff, Landrine, & Campbell, 2000). Belle and Doucet (2003) noted that these studies probably underestimate the degree of sex discrimination and its impact on depression in women, because discrimination is often continual and routinized, and many women are unaware of the discrimination they face daily. Ethnic minority women endure not only sex discrimination but also racial discrimination. Race discrimination has also been found to have negative consequences for women, including depression (U.S. Department of Health and Human Services, 2001).

Another form of sex discrimination is *sexual harassment*, defined as "unwelcome sexual advances, requests for sexual favors, or other verbal or physical conduct of a sexual nature" that either are a condition of employment or create an intimidating or hostile work environment (Gutek & Done, 2001, p. 368). Studies of community samples suggest that 35% to 50% of women, compared with 9% to 35% of men, have been sexually harassed at some point in their working lives, with higher estimates being found in male-dominated work settings (Gutek, 1985). Although sexist comments are the most common form of sexual harassment, 1% to 3% of women have been the victims of sexual coercion on the job (Barak, Pitterman, & Yitzhaki, 1995; Fitzgerald, Swan, & Magley, 1997). Experiences of sexual harassment are associated with both elevated depressive symptoms and an increased risk of major depression (Dansky & Kilpatrick, 1997; Fitzgerald et al., 1997). The full extent to which sexual harassment contributes to the gender difference in depression remains unknown.

Can the literature on acute and chronic stressors help us to understand why the gender difference in depression emerges in early adolescence? Rates of sexual abuse of girls increase substantially in early adolescence, potentially contributing to the increase in rates of depression in girls (Russell, 1984; although also see Finkelhor, Hotaling, Lewis, & Smith, 1990). Twenty-one percent of first rapes happen to girls under 12 years of age and another 32% happen to girls between 12 and 17 years (Tjaden & Thoennes, 1998). It is less clear that rates of chronic stressors, such as poverty or discrimination, increase in this time period. Several theorists have argued that girls' choices of activities and career paths, and their basic freedoms, are increasingly curtailed as they mature sexually in early adolescence (see Helgeson, 2000, for reviews). However, the extent to which the growing awareness of women's social roles and the burden of fear of sexual and physical abuse contributes to the increase in depression in girls during this period has not been established.

Gender Differences in Stress Reactivity

Several studies have suggested that following a stressful event, women are more likely than men to experience depression (Kessler & McLeod, 1984; Nazroo, Edwards, & Brown, 1997; Uhlenhuth & Paykel, 1973). For example, Maciejewski, Prigerson, and Mazure (2001) analyzed data from a nationwide community-based sample of 1,024 men and 1,800 women and found no gender differences in exposure to a number of stressful life events, but that women were approximately three times more likely than men to experience major depression in the wake of a stressful life event. Kessler and McLeod (1984) and Nazroo et al. (1997) found that the gender difference in depressive responses was particularly great for "network events"—events that happened to close friends and family members. They argued that women suffer a "cost of caring" because their deep emotional

others put them at risk for depression when negative
s befall others.

Other theorists suggest that women's greater tendency to react to stressors with depression compared with men is due to certain personality or cognitive characteristics, or certain biological vulnerabilities, which women carry more often than do men.

Cognitive-Personality Factors

Prominent psychological models of depression suggest that certain cognitive tendencies increase risk of depression, particularly when these tendencies interact with negative life events.

Negative cognitive styles. Beck and colleagues (Beck, Rush, Shaw, & Emery, 1979) argued that depression results from a negative cognitive triad in which individuals view themselves, the world, and the future in distorted and negative ways. Other cognitive theorists have focused on the attributions individuals make for events and have shown that people who attribute negative events to internal, stable, and global factors are at increased risk for depressive symptoms, particularly hopelessness symptoms (Abramson et al., 2002; Abramson, Metalsky, & Alloy, 1989; Abramson, Seligman, & Teasdale, 1978; Peterson & Seligman, 1984). Some studies have found that women are more likely than men to score high on measures of hopelessness and low on measures of perceived control (Angell et al., 1999; Hankin & Abramson, 2002; Nolen-Hoeksema, Larson, & Grayson, 1999), which then may contribute to more depressive symptoms in women than in men. However, studies using measures of the dysfunctional attitudes that Beck suggests are key to depression have found that men score higher than do women (Angell et al., 1999; Gotlib, 1984; Haeffel et al., 2003). Thus, the extent to which negative cognitive styles contribute to the gender difference in depression is unclear and may depend on which negative cognitive style is being measured.

Interpersonal dependency. Another cognitive-personality characteristic associated with depressive symptoms is excessive interpersonal dependency, also referred to as sociotropy (Beck,

1987; Clark, Beck, & Brown, 1992) or unmitigated communion (Helgeson, 1994). People high on this characteristic are excessively concerned with the opinions of others and about the security of their relationships with others, to the point of sacrificing their own needs to maintain relationships. Studies have shown that people high on sociotropy or unmitigated communion are more likely to have depressive symptoms or be diagnosed with depression (Clark et al., 1992; Hammen, 1999; Mazure, Bruce, Maciejewski, & Jacobs, 2000).

Women appear more likely than men to score high on some measures of sociotropy or unmitigated communion (Helgeson, 1994; Helgeson & Fritz, 1998; Leadbeater, Blatt, & Quinlan, 1995; Nolen-Hoeksema & Jackson, 2001; Spence, Helmreich, & Holahan, 1979). In addition, at least one study has found that unmitigated communion mediates the gender difference in depressive symptoms (Helgeson & Fritz, 1996).

Rumination. Rumination is the tendency to focus on one's symptoms of distress, and the possible causes and consequences of these symptoms, in a repetitive and passive manner rather than in an active, problem-solving manner (Nolen-Hoeksema, 2004). When people ruminate, they have thoughts such as, "Why am I so unmotivated? I just can't get going. I'm never going to get my work done feeling this way." Although some rumination may be a natural response to distress and depression, there are stable individual differences in the tendency to ruminate (Nolen-Hoeksema & Davis, 1999). People who ruminate a great deal in response to their sad or depressed moods have longer periods of depressive symptoms and are more likely to be diagnosed with major depressive disorder (Nolen-Hoeksema, 2004). The effects of rumination on depression over time remain significant even after baseline levels of depression are controlled for.

Women are more likely than men to ruminate in response to sad, depressed, or anxious moods (Nolen-Hoeksema, Larson, & Grayson, 1999; Tamres, Janicki, & Helgeson, 2002). The gender difference in rumination exists in both self-report survey and interview studies and in laboratory studies in which women's and men's responses to sad moods are observed (Butler & Nolen-Hoeksema, 1994). In turn, when gender differences in rumination are statistically controlled, the gender difference in depression becomes nonsignificant, which suggests that rumination helps to account for the gender difference in depressive symptoms (Nolen-Hoeksema et al., 1999).

How does rumination contribute to depression? Laboratory studies show that when people ruminate in response to a depressed mood, their memories of their past, their interpretations of the present, and their expectations for the future become more negative and distorted (Lyubomirsky, Caldwell, & Nolen-Hoeksema, 1998; Lyubomirsky & Nolen-Hoeksema, 1995). Thus, ruminators become increasingly negative and hopeless in their thinking and show many of the cognitive errors described by Beck (1987) as contributing to depression. Moreover, ruminators generate less effective solutions to solve their problems, and they are less confident about implementing these solutions (Lyubomirsky & Nolen-Hoeksema, 1995; Ward, Lyubomirsky, Sousa, & Nolen-Hoeksema, 2003). Thus, they are less likely to take positive action on their environment to overcome other factors contributing to their depression.

Cognitive-personality characteristics and the emergence of gender differences in depression. Several theorists have argued that the gender difference in interpersonal orientation increases substantially in early adolescence, around the time the gender difference in depression emerges (Helgeson, 2000; Leadbeater et al., 1995). Social forces pressure girls to become increasingly interpersonally oriented as they enter the dating world, where submissiveness to males is valued on the dating market and unmitigated communion is fostered (Helgeson, 2000). Cyranowski, Frank, Young, and Shear (2000) also suggested that the fact that girls can begin to bear children in adolescence triggers evolutionarily determined biological factors that enhance interpersonal orientation.

The existing evidence suggests that gender differences in rumination are present even before the gender differences in depression emerge in early adolescence (see Nolen-Hoeksema & Girgus, 1994). Differences in the socialization of boys and girls (Nolen-Hoeksema, 2004) likely contribute to this gender difference. Parents may be even more unlikely to teach their daughters than their sons problem-solving approaches to dealing with negative affect. Parents appear very concerned that their sons not express stereotypically feminine emotions, such as sadness or fear, and that they "be strong" and "act like a little man" when distressed (Maccoby & Jacklin, 1974). Sanctions against males displaying sadness continue in adulthood. Siegel and Alloy (1990) found that men with depression were evaluated much more negatively than were women with depression. These social reinforcements and punishments may motivate boys and men to develop active styles of responding to their depressed moods. At times, these active responses may be inappropriate (e.g., engaging in reckless behavior to avoid thinking about one's depressed mood), but much of the time, these active strategies may involve either positive distractions or constructive problem solving. Parents may not directly reinforce rumination in girls; they may simply fail to encourage active problem solving when girls are sad or upset. A tendency to ruminate may then interact with challenges of early adolescence that trigger initial depressive symptoms in girls to contribute to the increase in depression in girls relative to boys in early adolescence. Preventative interventions targeting rumination must start in childhood if they are to forestall the development of the gender difference in depression found in adolescence.

Biological Factors

Biological factors, as well as psychosocial factors, may contribute to greater rates of depression in women compared with men, both directly and indirectly, by increasing women's reactivity to stress.

Genetic factors. Family history studies clearly show that depression runs in families, particularly among female members, and twin studies confirm that genetics play a role in vulnerability to depression. Some twin studies of major depression suggest that genetics play a heavier role in this disorder for women than for men (Bierut et al., 1999; Jacobson & Rowe, 1999; Silberg et al., 1999). Other twin studies, however, have found no gender difference in the heritability of depression (Eaves et al., 1997; Kendler & Prescott, 1999; Rutter, Silberg, O'Connor, & Simonoff, 1999). Whether a gender difference in heritability is found seems to depend in part on how depression is operationalized. Two studies suggest that gender differences in the heritability of depression are found when relatively broad criteria are used, but not when more narrow criteria for depression are used (Bierut et al., 1999; Kendler, Gardner, Neale, & Prescott, 2001).

Other studies have suggested that the genes influencing the risk for major depression in women and men may not be the same (Bierut et al., 1999; Kendler et al., 2001). Zubenko and colleagues (2002a, 2002b) have used genetic linkage analyses to identify a specific candidate gene (*CREB1*) that may interact with estrogen receptors to contribute to higher rates of depression in women than in men. This gene plays a role in neuronal plasticity, cognition, and long-term memory, abnormalities of which commonly occur in people with major depression. Abnormalities in this gene were associated with unipolar mood disorders in female relatives of people with early-onset recurrent depression, but not in male relatives of people with this type of depression.

Gonadal hormones. Over the past 40 years, a vast literature on the relationship between gonadal hormones (particularly estrogen and progesterone) and mood in women has developed (see reviews by Steiner, 1992; Steiner & Dunn, 1996; Steiner, Dunn, & Born, 2003). At the heart of this literature is the observation that some women develop depression, or experience severe exacerbation of an existing depression, during periods when hormone levels change substantially, including during the premenstrual (or late luteal) phase of the menstrual cycle, during the postpartum period, and at the start of menopause (Seeman, 1997; Steiner et al., 2003).

Sufficient evidence has not been found to suggest a simple direct relationship between hormonal levels and depression. Researchers have not found consistent differences in levels of estrogen or progesterone between women with premenstrual dysphoric disorder (PMDD) and women who have no experience of this disorder. Further, most women with PMDD appear to have normal ovarian functioning (Steiner et al., 2003). None-theless, PMDD is, by definition, a disorder marked by a period of clear changes in hormones.

Recent studies found an increased likelihood of depressive symptoms among women during the transition to menopause and a decreased likelihood after menopause, after adjustment for other predictors of depression (Bromberger et al., 2001; Free-man et al., 2004; Maartens, Knottnerus, & Pop, 2002). It is impor-tant to note that most women do *not* experience significant mood changes during these periods. Yet, a small subset of women, particularly women with a family history of depression or a personal history of previous depressive episodes, do experience significant increases in core depressive symptoms at these times (Nolen-Hoeksema, 2002).

Steiner et al. (2003) proposed that in women with certain un-derlying vulnerabilities (particularly a genetic vulnerability to depression, but perhaps also vulnerabilities due to psychosocial stressors and trauma), fluctuations in gonadal hormones cause dysregulation in the neurotransmitters that regulate mood, par-ticularly serotonin, leading to depression. Steiner et al. reviewed the substantial evidence that gonadal hormones and neuro-transmitters have many reciprocal effects on each other. They then described a variety of mechanisms by which hormone–neurotransmitter interactions could explain depressions associ-ated with hormonal change in puberty, the premenstrual period, postpartum period, and menopause. For example, recent studies suggest that women with PMDD have elevated levels of serum testosterone in the luteal phase compared with control partici-pants, which may contribute to the symptom of irritability (Eriks-son, Alling, & Andersch, 1994; Eriksson, Sundblad, & Lisjo, 1992). The elevated androgen levels in women with PMDD may inhibit serotonin levels, contributing to irritability and perhaps other symptoms of depression (Eriksson, Sundblad, Landen, & Steiner, 2000). Increasing serotonin availability through the use of selective serotonin reuptake inhibitors reduces irritability and depression.

Biological stress reactivity. Several biological factors may lead women to be more likely than men to have a dysregulated response to stress, which makes them more likely to develop depression secondary to stress (Weiss et al., 1999). Three key components of the neuroendocrine system—the hypothalamus, pituitary, and adrenal cortex—work together in response to stress in a feedback system that is richly interconnected with the limbic system and the cerebral cortex. This system is often referred to as the hypothalamic–pituitary–adrenal axis, or HPA axis. When humans are confronted with a stressor, the HPA axis normally becomes more active, increasing levels of hormones such as cortisol, which help the body to respond to the stressor by making it possible to fight the stressor or flee from it. Once the stressor is gone, the HPA axis returns to homeostasis.

People with depression tend to show chronic hyperactivity in the HPA axis and an inability of the HPA axis to return to normal functioning following a stressor (Young & Korszun, 1999). In turn, the excess hormones produced by heightened HPA activity seem to have an inhibiting effect on receptors for the monoamines. One model for the development of depression is that people exposed to chronic stress may develop poorly regulated neuroendocrine systems. Then, when they are exposed even to minor stressors later in life, the HPA axis overreacts and does not easily return to homeostasis, creating change in the functioning of the monoamine neurotransmitters in the brain, and an episode of depression is likely to ensue (Weiss, 1991).

Genetic factors may contribute to greater biological stress reactivity in women compared with men. For example, Zubenko and colleagues (2002a, 2002b) suggested that alterations in the gene they have linked to depression in women but not in men (i.e., CREB1) may lead to more depression in women because it reduces their resilience to environmental stress. (For further evidence of genetic moderators of the stress response, see Caspi et al. [2003].)

Changes in the hormonal milieu may also increase stress reactivity in these women (Young & Korszun, 1999). The ovarian hormones modulate the regulation of the HPA axis, which plays an important role in stress responses (Steiner et al., 2003). Some women may have depressions during periods of rapid change in levels of ovarian hormones (the postpartum period, premenstrual period, perimenopause, and puberty) because hormonal changes may trigger dysregulation of the stress response, making these women more vulnerable to depression, particularly when they are confronted with stress. For example, some studies of pubertal children have shown that primarily the girls who are confronted by major stressors (such as their parents' divorce) at the time of peak pubertal and hormonal changes are most likely to show increases in distress (Angold, Worthman, & Costello, 1997; Brooks-Gunn & Warren, 1989; Steiner, Born, & Martin, 2000).

Intriguing new animal research by Shors and colleagues (Shors & Leuner, 2003) provides some clues as to how changes in the stress response due to changes in hormone levels may contribute to depression in women (see also Young, Midgley, Carlson, & Brown, 2000). Using animal models, they found that females with high levels of estrogen resulting from normal fluctuations or chemical intervention showed significantly impaired performance in an inescapable-stress, conditioned-response paradigm, whereas estrogen levels have no effects on males' performance (Wood & Shors, 1998). The inability to perform even simple responses when confronted by stressors may increase females' stress reactivity. Moreover, previous experiences with inescapable stressors elevate estrogen levels in females and impair anatomical measures of plasticity in brain regions associated with emotion and memory function (Shors, Pickett, Wood, & Paczynski, 1999). More recent animal studies by Shansky et al. (2004) show that estrogen amplifies the stress response in the prefrontal cortex, which may increase susceptibility to stress-related disorders. Taken together, these results suggest that exposure to stressful experiences enhances estrogen beyond normal circulating levels in females, altering synaptic plasticity in limbic brain regions associated with emotion, thereby dampening affect and performance in response to challenges. This model is preliminary but, if replicated in humans, could reveal important links between the stressful experiences, hormonal functioning, stress reactivity, and vulnerability to depression in the small number of women with hormonally related depressions.

Women may be more likely to have a dysregulated HPA response because they are more likely than men to have experienced traumatic events during childhood, which in turn negatively affect the development of the biological stress response (see Weiss et al., 1999). Studies of animals and humans suggest that early, severe stressors, such as sexual or physical abuse during childhood, can lead to dysregulation in biological responses to stress, as measured by cortisol levels, adrenocorticotropic hormone levels, and cardiac measures, which persist into adulthood (Graham, Heim, Goodman, Miller, & Nemeroff, 1999; Heim & Nemeroff, 2001; Heim et al., 2000; Zahn-Waxler, 2000). Women who were sexually abused as children and who are retraumatized as adults show even greater neuroendocrine stress reactivity (Heim et al., 2002).

An Integrative Model

Each of the factors discussed in this chapter—being sexually or physically assaulted or facing ongoing abuse, living in unrelenting poverty, being the victim of discrimination, having a negative cognitive style, being excessively dependent on others, being a ruminator, or having genetic vulnerabilities, hormonal changes, and HPA axis dysregulation—could independently contribute to women's higher rates of depression compared with men. These factors likely interact in complex ways to produce depression, however, particularly in women (see Figure 1.1).

As noted earlier, the stressful experiences more common in women's lives than men's lives, including acute sexual traumas and chronic strains such as poverty, can cause biological changes that increase women's stress reactivity (see Weiss et al., 1999). Genetic vulnerability to depression, or to dysregulation of neuroendocrine or neurotransmitter systems, could further enhance the negative effects of early stressors on these systems (Kendler, 1998).

Dysregulation of the biological stress response could contribute to new episodes of depression both through biological mechanisms (e.g., by affecting serotonergic systems) and by affecting a woman's behavioral response to new stressors. If a woman is less effective in responding to these new stressors, the stressors might become chronic or may have long-term consequences for her quality of life (e.g., she may quit a stressful job, which leads to severe reductions in her income).

Stressful experiences could also increase psychosocial vulnerability to depression in women by exacerbating a preexisting

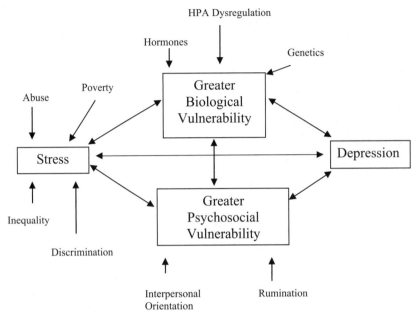

Figure 1.1.   An integrative model. HPA = hypothalmic–
pituitary–adrenal.

tendency to ruminate and by contributing to the development
of interpersonal dependency or negative cognitive styles. One
study found that women with histories of sexual abuse were
more prone to ruminate, possibly because they were vigilant for
signs of threat and danger in their lives or were still trying to
reconcile their abuse experiences with their views of the world
and themselves (Nolen-Hoeksema, 1998). In addition, women
who face constant daily strain from lack of equity in their relationships, lack of appreciation at work and at home, and lack of
financial resources are more prone to ruminate and to have
negative cognitive styles (Nolen-Hoeksema et al., 1999). Rose
and Abramson (1992) suggested that emotional abuse may be
a particularly important predictor of adult cognitive risk for
depression because, by definition, the abuser supplies negative
cognitions to the abused in the process of delivering the abuse.
Others (Gibb et al., 2001; Maciejewski & Mazure, in press) subse-
quently found that negative cognitive style appears to mediate
the relationship between early emotional abuse and adult depression. As Maciejewski and Mazure (in press) have pointed out,

early traumatic emotional experience appears to lead to the formation of negative cognitive styles that then confer life-long risk for depression, particularly in the face of subsequent stress.

Rumination unfortunately may then make it even more difficult for these women to assimilate their experiences cognitively and to take action to overcome their negative environments. People who ruminate have more difficulty making sense of traumatic experiences in terms of their philosophical or religious views, which helps to perpetuate their depressions (Nolen-Hoeksema & Larson, 1999). As noted earlier, people who ruminate also have more difficulty generating effective solutions to complex interpersonal problems and are less motivated and confident in implementing the solutions they do generate. Thus, stressful experiences may contribute to more rumination in women and, in turn, rumination may help to perpetuate the stress in women's life (see Nolen-Hoeksema et al., 1999, for evidence supporting these reciprocal effects). For example, women who are married to emotionally abusive partners and who ruminate about their situations may have more trouble seeing existing opportunities to leave the marriage and rebuild their lives.

In a similar way, the behaviors motivated by interpersonal dependency can contribute to more stress (Joiner & Coyne, 1999). People who take on the pain of others may live with more stress than do those who do not, and those who rely on others for their self-esteem often require excessive assurances of love, which leads to mood swings when reassurance is not forthcoming, or leads to alienation and rejection by friends and family, who tire of their high need for social support. In one study, adolescents who scored high on interpersonal dependency reported more interpersonal stressors, and these interpersonal stressors accounted for the increase in psychological distress over a 4-month period (Helgeson & Fritz, 1996). In a daily diary study of college students, people who scored high on interpersonal dependency were more adversely affected by interpersonal conflict than were those who scored low on unmitigated communion (Reynolds et al., in press).

Hammen (2003) made the critical point that depression generates its own stress. Depressed women are more likely than nondepressed women to report stressful events to which they had contributed, especially interpersonal conflicts and other interpersonal events. Observational studies also show that depression can generate interpersonal stress. For example, depressed women have lower quality interactions and communications with their children, even though they may fervently desire to be good mothers (Hammen, 2003). The problems these women show in parenting may be a direct result of their symptoms of depression, such as irritability, apathy, and poor concentration. Finally, some of the parenting problems of depressed mothers may actually be due to high levels of stress in their lives (e.g., lack of money, ongoing abuse) as much as to depression per se.

Depression also probably has effects on both the biological and the psychological factors that contribute to greater stress reactivity in women, as shown in Figure 1.1. Latent negative cognitions, of which individuals are not consciously aware, are more easily primed and brought to awareness by sad mood inductions in people with a history of depression than in people with no history of depression (Teasdale, 1988; Teasdale & Dent, 1987). For example, one study found no differences between formerly depressed participants and nondepressed participants in negative, self-defeating cognitions when both groups were in a neutral mood. But after a sad mood induction, the formerly depressed participants voiced significantly more negative cognitions than did the never depressed participants (Miranda & Persons, 1988).

Negative mood can prime the negative cognitions of depression that tend to be woven together in associative networks. Each depressive episode may strengthen the connections between the nodes in these networks, making it easier for an incipient depressive mood to activate the entire network. In addition, the relevant stressors associated with each new experience of depression may more easily prime and bring to awareness content themes within the network (e.g., concerns over social relationships). Finally, awareness of these negative cognitions and concerns could lead to an upswell in ruminative thinking.

Early adolescence is a time during which many of the social and psychological factors illustrated in the figure may also lead to changes for girls, as has been discussed throughout this chapter (see Nolen-Hoeksema & Girgus, 1994). During this period, when girls are developing secondary sex characteristics, rates of all types of sexual abuse against girls increase substantially (Russell, 1984). These experiences of abuse thus could contribute directly to increases in rates of depression in girls. Helgeson (2000) argued that during early adolescence, girls also become aware of the limitations on their choices of activities and careers imposed by societal gender roles, and the pressures for them to become submissive to males. This awareness leads girls to suppress their desires and assertive behaviors and to become more interpersonally oriented, which in turn lowers their well-being. An interpersonal orientation may interact with the challenges of negotiating the world of heterosexual relationships, which begin in early adolescence, contributing to the increase in depression in some girls. A greater tendency to ruminate in girls may similarly interact with increases in distress-inducing stressors in adolescence to increase rates of depression in girls during this period (Nolen-Hoeksema & Girgus, 1994).

Biological factors may also interact with each other and with psychosocial stressors in early adolescence to contribute to the emergence of gender differences in depression. Steiner et al. (2000) noted that the hormonal changes of puberty may trigger a previously latent genetic vulnerability in girls. For example, the influx of high levels of estrogen and progesterone in puberty may trigger a genetic vulnerability to dysregulation of neurotransmitter systems or the HPA axis, causing these girls to have biological tendencies to poorly regulated stress responses. In addition, as already reviewed, the hormonal changes of puberty may interact with stressors during this same period to increase girls' rates of depression relative to rates for boys.

Recommendations for Research

A number of recommendations for future research are suggested by the integrative model just proposed and by the review of existing research.

1. *Improve the operationalization of depression and related constructs.* Imprecision and inconsistency in the measurement of depression and of possible etiological factors have hampered the ability to draw conclusions about any of the potential contributors to the gender difference in depression. For example, the literature on abuse finds very different prevalence rates from study to study depending on the definition and measurement of abuse. How central constructs are defined and measured also affects the observed relationships between abuse and depression. In a similar way, various studies of poverty, economic inequalities, and discrimination have defined and operationalized these constructs differently (Belle & Doucet, 2003), thus affecting the observed relationships to depression and other psychological variables.

Bierut (2000) also noted that a critical methodological advance in studies of the genetics of the gender difference in depression will be in the standardization of depression across studies. In Bierut et al.'s (1999) study of twins, estimates of the significance of gender differences in the heritability of depression varied with the diagnostic criteria for depression used, but not in ways that could illuminate when gender differences are or are not likely to be found. In addition, there are likely to be real differences in the heritability, or in the contribution of other biological factors, to different forms of depression (e.g., major depressive disorder vs. dysthymic disorder vs. adjustment disorder with depressed mood), and it is critical that studies not combine people with these different forms of depression simply to increase the available sample size.

2. *Encourage or require gender difference analyses in studies of depression.* If investigators do not include both women and men in their samples or do not routinely examine gender differences in their data, the contribution of a proposed etiological factor to the gender difference in depression remains unknown. For example, much of the literature on sexual abuse includes only samples of women, making it impossible to compare the relative contribution of abuse to depression in women versus the same in men. In a similar way, a major problem in using much of the biological literature to draw conclusions about the role of

biological factors in producing the gender differences in depression is that most studies are not designed to investigate gender differences. Instead, these studies often have largely female participants and thus can draw conclusions only about the role of a given biological factor in depression in women. Showing that hormones, HPA axis dysregulation, or genes contribute to depression in women tells little about whether these factors significantly account for women's much greater rates of depression compared with men. It will be important for future studies to include both male and female samples and to test directly whether a given biological factor accounts for a significant portion of the difference in rates of depression between men and women in that sample.

3. *Conduct longitudinal studies.* Most of the research used to support claims that a particular factor contributes to the gender difference in depression has been cross-sectional. For example, most studies of the relationships between depression and poverty or other chronic stressors are cross-sectional and thus cannot determine cause versus consequence. It is highly likely that depression and stress have reciprocal effects on each other, as Hammen (2003) argued. The symptoms of depression make it difficult for people to function optimally, leading to new stressors in individuals' lives, such as the loss of a job. Ongoing abuse is particularly potent in maintaining depressive symptom severity (Campbell & Soeken, 1999). Once a battered woman is away from the abusive environment, her symptoms often decrease (Astin, Lawrence, & Foy, 1993; Campbell, Sullivan, & Davidson, 1995). Modeling the reciprocal effects of stress and depression on each other is difficult but essential for a full understanding of the disorder.

4. *Take a life span developmental approach and focus depression research on times of high risk in women's lives.* Understanding why gender differences in depression develop in early adolescence will be critical to the development of preventative intervention programs. Understanding why some women experience more depression during the postpartum period and perimenopause will help in identifying targets for interventions among women at high risk. These periods of risk for depression in women's lives also represent a natural laboratory for the study of depression,

potentially affording more statistical power to identify etiological factors, because the prevalence of episodes of depression in certain women will be higher during these periods.

5. *Conduct interdisciplinary research.* It is clear that psychological, social, and biological factors interact to produce the gender differences in depression. An understanding of this phenomenon will advance when researchers move away from examining one possible contributor to women's depressions at a time and begin to test integrated models with interdisciplinary techniques.

6. *Keep contextual factors in focus in all types of research.* The contextual realities of women's lives, especially their lower social power and particular social roles, influence every aspect of their functioning, including their biological and psychological functioning. It will be important to keep these contextual realities in mind in studies of any potential contributor to the gender difference in depression. In addition, there are wide variations among women due to differences in ethnicity and cultural background, socioeconomic status, and membership in other social categories, which may affect both the presence of risk factors for depression and the relationship of these risk factors to depression. Future research should focus more on understanding how variations across groups of women contribute to their high rates of depression.

Recommendations for Policy

1. *Use current knowledge about the contributors to the gender difference in depression to design screening, prevention, and intervention programs for girls and women.* Although much more research is needed on the etiology of gender differences in depression, sufficient knowledge exists to target certain groups of women for screening, prevention, and intervention programs. For example, such programs should focus on girls in early adolescence and women who are pregnant, postpartum, or perimenopausal and have a history of previous depression.

Because early sexual abuse appears to be a potent contributor to depression in women, sexually abused women are an important target for screening, prevention, and intervention programs for depression. Koss and colleagues (2003) argued that the symptoms of depression and the diagnostic criteria for depressive disorders may better reflect the range of responses of abuse victims than do the symptoms and criteria for posttraumatic stress disorder (PTSD), particularly for women who are repeatedly abused, such as incest victims and victims of male partner violence. These women often ruminate a lot about the causes of their abuse as well as experience changes in their core beliefs about the self and the world as manifest through maladaptive cognitive styles, and many experience social, spiritual, and physical health changes.

Refocusing attention for abuse victims on symptoms of depression rather than PTSD alone could have important clinical implications. The vast majority of abuse victims seek help from their primary care physicians rather than mental health specialists, if they seek any help at all (Koss, Ingram, & Pepper, 1997; Koss, Woodruff, & Koss, 1991). The American Medical Association issued guidelines in 1992 that encouraged physicians to screen for experiences of abuse in their patients and provide treatment for the psychological as well as physical consequences of abuse, but the available data suggest that primary care providers rarely ask their patients about their abuse experiences (Koss et al., 1997; Ruddy & McDaniel, 1995). Although educational efforts alone have shown little effect on increasing the identification of exposure to violence, systems approaches have proven more effective. A combination of training, clinical protocols, availability of support services to respond when cases are identified, chart reviews, communication of screening rates by departments, and posters and reminder cards throughout clinics has both increased the rate of screening by providers and communicated to patients that providers are responsive to these problems (Salber & McCaw, 2000). Koss et al. (2003) suggested that physicians may be better equipped and more comfortable in screening for violence and treating depression than they are for screening for victimization and treating PTSD.

Helgeson (2000) argued that identifying those young women who are turning from interests in personal activities and achievements to an overconcern with others, and then helping them to reclaim their own interests and independent sources of self-esteem, will reduce excessive interpersonal dependency in these women and lower their risk of depression. The literature on gender differences in rumination and depression suggests that explicit training in nonruminative responses to one's mood swings is an important component of therapy for women who are depressed. Therapy with women could emphasize empowerment and building skills in active problem solving to overcome rumination and depression.

2. *Encourage social programs that reduce the prevalence of the social contributors to depression in women.* More effort needs to be made at a societal level to prevent the high rates of abuse, poverty, and other stressors in women's lives. Belle and Doucet (2003) emphasized the need to raise the living standard for women by ensuring that poor women get the resources to which they are entitled (Belle & Doucet, 2003). Belle and Doucet further argued that reducing the enormous disparities between rich and poor will change attitudes toward the poor, lessening the impact of lower income on their well-being.

3. *Develop prevention and intervention programs that address the multiple contributors to depression in women.* The reciprocal relationships among the variables shown in Figure 1.1 suggest that no one variable or vulnerability factor should be the sole focus of interventions, and underscore the importance of a holistic approach that addresses as many of these vulnerability factors as possible. Thus, interventions with depressed women need to attend to their past and current history of severe stressors, their psychological and biological reactivity to stress, and the effects of their depression on their environment and reactivity.

Such holistic approaches require collaborations between psychiatrists who specialize in biological treatments and psychotherapists who can help depressed women learn more adaptive coping and interpersonal skills and deal with the major stressors in their lives. In addition, continued political action aimed at reducing the incidence of stressors associated with women's social status and roles will be critical to reducing the overall rates of depression in women.

4. *Educate the public on the risk factors for depression in women.* In particular, help both the lay public and health care professionals understand the multiple contributors to depression in women,

so as to increase their understanding of the need for holistic approaches to prevention and treatment of depression in women. Stigma remains an obstacle in reducing the number of individuals who seek treatment for depression. The public needs to be provided with continued education campaigns, empirically designed to be maximally effective, to help them recognize symptoms and engage in treatment.

References

Abramson, L. Y., Alloy, L. B., Hankin, B. L., Haeffel, G. J., MacCoon, D. G., & Gibb, B. E. (2002). Cognitive vulnerability-stress models of depression in a self-regulatory and psychobiological context. In I. H. Gotlib & C. L. Hammen (Eds.), *Handbook of depression* (pp. 268–294). New York: Guilford Press.

Abramson, L. Y., Metalsky, G. I., & Alloy, L. B. (1989). Hopelessness depression: A theory-based subtype of depression. *Psychological Review, 96,* 358–372.

Abramson, L. Y., Seligman, M. E. P., & Teasdale, J. (1978). Learned helplessness in humans: Critique and reformulation. *Journal of Abnormal Psychology, 87,* 49–74.

Angell, K. E., Abramson, L. Y., Alloy, L. B., Hankin, B. L., Hogan, M. E., Whitehouse, W. G., & Hyde, J. S. (1999, November). *Gender differences in dysphoria and etiological factors: Ethnic variations.* Paper presented at the meeting of the Association for Advancement of Behavior Therapy, Toronto, Ontario, Canada.

Angold, A., Costello, E., & Worthman, C. (1998). Puberty and depression: The roles of age, pubertal status, and pubertal timing. *Psychological Medicine, 28,* 51–61.

Angold, A., Worthman, C., & Costello, E. (1997, February). *Puberty and depression: A longitudinal epidemiological diagnostic study.* Paper presented at the annual meeting of the American Psychopathological Association, New York.

Astin, M. C., Lawrence, K. J., & Foy, D. W. (1993). Posttraumatic stress disorder among battered women: Risk and resiliency factors. *Violence and Victims, 8,* 17–28.

Barak, A., Pitterman, Y., & Yitzhaki, R. (1995). An empirical test of the role of power differential in originating sexual harassment. *Basic and Applied Social Psychology, 17,* 497–518.

Bassuk, E., Buckner, J., Perloff, J., & Bassuk, S. (1998). Prevalence of mental health and substance use disorders among homeless and low-income housed mothers. *American Journal of Psychiatry, 155,* 1561–1564.

Bebbington, P. E., Tennant, C., & Hurry, J. (1991). Adversity in groups with an increased risk of minor affective disorder. *British Journal of Psychiatry, 158*, 33–48.

Beck, A. T. (1987). Cognitive models of depression. *Journal of Cognitive Psychotherapy: An International Quarterly, 1*, 5–37.

Beck, A. T., Rush, A. J., Shaw, B. F., & Emery, G. (1979). *Cognitive therapy of depression.* New York: Guilford Press.

Belle, D., & Doucet, J. (2003). Poverty, inequality, and discrimination as sources of depression among U.S. women. *Psychology of Women Quarterly, 27*, 101–113.

Belle, D., Longfellow, C., & Makosky, V. (1982). Stress, depression and the mother–child relationship: Report of a field study. *International Journal of Sociology of the Family, 12*, 251–263.

Bierut, L. (2000, October). *Genetic contributions to the development of depression: Are there gender differences?* Paper presented at the American Psychological Association Summit 2000 on Women and Depression, Queenstown, MD.

Bierut, L. J., Heath, A. C., Bucholz, K. K., Dinwiddie, S. H., Madden, P. A. F., Statham, D. J., et al. (1999). Major depressive disorder in a community-based twin sample: Are there different genetic and environmental contributions for men and women? *Archives of General Psychiatry, 57*, 557–563.

Bromberger, J. T., Meyer, P. M., Kravitz, H. M., Sommer, B., Cordal, A., Powell, L., et al. (2001). Psychologic distress and natural menopause: A multiethnic community study. *American Journal of Public Health, 91*, 1435–1442.

Brooks-Gunn, J., & Warren, M. P. (1989). Biological and social contributions to negative affect in young adolescent girls. *Child Development, 60*, 40–55.

Brown, G. W., & Birley, J. L. T. (1968). Crises and life changes and the onset of schizophrenia. *Journal of Health and Social Behavior, 9*, 203–214.

Brown, G. W., & Harris, T. O. (1978). *Social origins of depression: A study of psychiatric disorder in women.* New York: Free Press.

Brown, G. W., & Moran, P. (1997). Single mothers, poverty and depression. *Psychological Medicine, 27*, 21–33.

Bruce, M. L., Takeuchi, D., & Leaf, P. (1991). Poverty and psychiatric status. *Archives of General Psychiatry, 48*, 470–474.

Butler, L. D., & Nolen-Hoeksema, S. (1994). Gender differences in responses to a depressed mood in a college sample. *Sex Roles, 30*, 331–346.

Campbell, J. C., & Soeken, K. L. (1999). Women's responses to battering: A test of the model. *Research in Nursing & Health, 22*, 49–58.

Campbell, R., Sullivan, C. M., & Davidson, W. S. (1995). Women who use domestic violence shelters: Changes in depression over time. *Psychology of Women Quarterly, 19*, 237–255.

Caspi, A., Sugden, K., Moffitt, T. E., Taylor, A., Craig, I. W., Harrington, H. L., et al. (2003, July 18). Influence of life stress on depression: Moderation by a polymorphism in the 5-HTT gene. *Science, 301*, 386–389.

Clark, D., Beck, A., & Brown, G. (1992). Sociotropy, autonomy, and life event perceptions in dysphoric and non dysphoric individuals. *Cognitive Therapy and Research, 16,* 635–652.

Cyranowski, J. M., Frank, E., Young, E., & Shear, K. (2000). Adolescent onset of the gender difference in lifetime rates of major depression. *Archives of General Psychiatry, 57,* 21–27.

Dansky, B. S., & Kilpatrick, D. G. (1997). Effects of sexual harassment. In W. O'Donohue (Ed.), *Sexual harassment: Theory, research, treatment* (pp. 152–174). Boston: Allyn & Bacon.

Dube, S. R., Anda, R. F., Felitti, V. J., Chapman, D. P., Williamson, D. F., & Giles, W. H. (2001, December 26). Child abuse, household dysfunction, and the risk of attempted suicide throughout the life span: Findings from the adverse childhood experiences study. *Journal of the American Medical Association, 286,* 3089–3096.

Eaton, W., Anthony, J., Gallo, J., Cai, G., Tien, A., Romanoski, A., et al. (1997). Natural history of Diagnostic Interview Schedule/DSM–IV Major Depression. *Archives of General Psychiatry, 54,* 993–999.

Eaton, W., & Muntaner, C. (1999). Socioeconomic stratification and mental disorder. In A. V. Horwitz & T. L. Scheid (Eds.), *A handbook for the study of mental health: Social contexts, theories and systems* (pp. 259–283). New York: Cambridge University Press.

Eaves, L. J., Silberg, J. L., Meyer, J. M., Maes, H. H., Simonoff, E., Pickles, A., et al. (1997). Genetics and developmental psychopathology: The main effects of genes and environment on behavioral problems in the Virginia twin study of adolescent behavioral development. *Journal of Child Psychology and Psychiatry, 38,* 965–980.

Eriksson, E., Alling, C., & Andersch, B. (1994). Cerebrospinal fluid levels of monoamine metabolites. A preliminary study of their relation to menstrual cycle phase, sex steroids, and pituitary hormones in healthy women and in women with premenstrual syndrome. *Neuropsychopharmacist, 11,* 201–213.

Eriksson, E., Sundblad, C., Landen, M., & Steiner, M. (2000). Behavioural effects of androgens in women. In M. Steiner, K. Yonkers, & E. Eriksson (Eds.), *Disorders in women* (pp. 233–246). London: Martin Dunitz.

Eriksson, E., Sundblad, C., & Lisjo, P. (1992). Serum levels of androgens are higher in women with premenstrual irritability and dysphoria than in controls. *Psychoneuroendocrinology, 17,* 195–204.

Feagin, J., & Feagin, C. (1978). *Discrimination American style: Institutional racism and sexism.* Englewood Cliffs, NJ: Prentice-Hall.

Finkelhor, D., Hotaling, G., Lewis, I. A., & Smith, C. (1990). Sexual abuse in a national survey of adult men and women: Prevalence, characteristics, and risk factors. *Child Abuse & Neglect, 14,* 19–28.

Fitzgerald, L. F., Swan, S., & Magley, V. J. (1997). But was it really sexual harassment? Legal, behavioral, and psychological definitions of the workplace victimization of women. In W. O'Donohue (Ed.), *Sexual harassment: Theory, research, treatment* (pp. 5–28). Boston: Allyn & Bacon.

Freeman, E. W., Sammel, M. D., Liu, L., Gracia, C. R., Nelson, D. B., & Holladner, L. (2004). Hormones and menopausal status as predictors of depression in women in transition to menopause. *Archives of General Psychiatry, 61,* 62–70.

Gibb, B. E., Alloy, L. B., Abramson, L. Y., Rose, D. T., Whitehouse, W. G., Donovan, P., et al. (2001). History of childhood maltreatment, negative cognitive styles, and episodes of depression in adulthood. *Cognitive Therapy and Research, 25,* 425–446.

Golding, J. (1999). Intimate partner violence as a risk factor for mental disorders: A meta-analysis. *Journal of Family Violence, 14,* 99–132.

Gotlib, I. H. (1984). Depression and general psychopathology in university students. *Journal of Abnormal Psychology, 93,* 19–30.

Graham, Y. P., Heim, C., Goodman, S. H., Miller, A. H., & Nemeroff, C. B. (1999). The effects of neonatal stress on brain development: Implications for psychopathology. *Development and Psychopathology, 11,* 545–565.

Gutek, B. A. (1985). *Sex and the workplace.* San Francisco: Jossey-Bass.

Gutek, B. A., & Done, R. S. (2001). Sexual harassment. In R. K. Unger (Ed.), *Handbook of the psychology of women and gender* (pp. 367–387). New York: Wiley.

Haeffel, G. J., Abramson, L. Y., Voelz, Z. R., Metalsky, G. I., Halberstadt, L., Dykman, B. M., et al. (2003). Cognitive vulnerability to depression and lifetime history of Axis I psychopathology: A comparison of negative cognitive styles (CSQ) and dysfunctional attitudes (DAS). *Journal of Cognitive Psychotherapy, 17,* 3–22.

Hammen, C. (1999). The emergence of an interpersonal approach to depression. In T. Joiner & J. Coyne (Eds.), *The interactional nature of depression: Advances in interpersonal approaches* (pp. 21–35). Washington, DC: American Psychological Association.

Hammen, C. (2003). Interpersonal stress and depression in women. *Journal of Affective Disorders, 74,* 49–57.

Hankin, B. L., & Abramson, L. Y. (2002). Measuring cognitive vulnerability to depression in adolescence: Reliability, validity, and gender differences. *Journal of Clinical Child and Adolescent Psychology, 31,* 491–504.

Heim, C., & Nemeroff, C. B. (2001). The role of childhood trauma in the neurobiology of mood and anxiety disorders: Preclinical and clinical studies. *Biological Psychiatry, 49,* 1023–1039.

Heim, C., Newport, J., Heit, S., Graham, Y., Wilcox, M., Bonsall, R., et al. (2000, August 2). Pituitary-adrenal and autonomic responses to stress in women after sexual and physical abuse in childhood. *Journal of the American Medical Association, 284,* 592–596.

Heim, C., Newport, D. J., Wagner, D., Wilcox, M. M., Miller, A. H., & Nemeroff, C. B. (2002). The role of early adverse experience and adulthood stress in the prediction of neuroendocrine stress reactivity in women: A multiple regression analysis. *Depression and Anxiety, 15,* 117–125.

Helgeson, V. (1994). Relation of agency and communion to well-being: Evidence and potential explanations. *Psychological Bulletin, 116,* 412–428.

Helgeson, V. (2000, October). *Psychosocial and cultural contributions to depression in women.* Paper presented at the American Psychological Association Summit 2000 on Women and Depression, Queenstown, MD.

Helgeson, V., & Fritz, H. (1996). Implications of communion and unmitigated communion for adolescent adjustment to Type I diabetes. *Women's Health: Research on Gender, Behavior, and Policy, 2,* 169–194.

Helgeson, V., & Fritz, H. (1998). A theory of unmitigated communion. *Personality and Social Psychology Review, 2,* 173–183.

Jacobson, K. C., & Rowe, D. C. (1999). Genetic and environmental influences on the relationships between family connectedness, school connectedness, and adolescent depressed mood: Sex differences. *Developmental Psychology, 35,* 926–939.

Joiner, T., & Coyne, J. C. (1999). *The interactional nature of depression: Advances in interpersonal approaches.* Washington, DC: American Psychological Association.

Keller, M., & Shapiro, R. (1981). Major depressive disorder: Initial results from a one-year prospective naturalistic follow-up study. *Journal of Nervous Mental Disorders, 169,* 761–768.

Kendler, K. (1998). Major depression and the environment: A psychiatric genetic perspective. *Pharmacopsychiatry, 31,* 5–9.

Kendler, K. S., Gardner, C. O., Neale, M. C., & Prescott, C. A. (2001). Genetic risk factors for major depression in men and women: Similar or different heritabilities and same or partly distinct genes? *Psychological Medicine, 31,* 605–616.

Kendler, K. S., & Prescott, C. A. (1999). A population based twin study of lifetime major depression in men and women. *Archives of General Psychiatry, 56,* 39–44.

Kessler, R. C., McGonagle, K. A., Swartz, M., Blazer, D. G., & Nelson, C. B. (1993). Sex and depression in the National Comorbidity Survey I: Lifetime prevalence, chronicity, and recurrence. *Journal of Affective Disorders, 29,* 85–96.

Kessler, R., & McLeod, J. (1984). Sex differences in vulnerability to undesirable life events. *American Sociological Review, 49,* 620–631.

Klonoff, E., Landrine, H., & Campbell, B. (2000). Sexist discrimination may account for well-known gender differences in psychiatric symptoms. *Psychology of Women Quarterly, 24,* 93–99.

Koss, M. P., Bailey, J., Yuan, N. P., Herrera, V. M., & Lichter, E. L. (2003). Depression and PTSD in survivors of male violence: Research and training initiatives to facilitate recovery. *Psychology of Women Quarterly, 27,* 130–142.

Koss, M. P., Ingram, M., & Pepper, S. (1997). Psychotherapists' role in the medical response to male-partner violence. *Psychotherapy, 34,* 386–396.

Koss, M. P., Woodruff, W. J., & Koss, P. G. (1991). Relation of criminal victimization to health perceptions among women medical patients. *Journal of Consulting and Clinical Psychology, 58,* 147–152.

Kovacs, M., Obrosky, D. S., & Sherrill, J. (2003). Developmental changes in the phenomenology of depression in girls compared to boys from childhood onward. *Journal of Affective Disorders, 74,* 33–48.

Landrine, H., Klonoff, E., Gibbs, J., Maning, V., & Lund, M. (1995). Physical and psychiatric correlates of gender discrimination: An application of the schedule of sexist events. *Psychology of Women Quarterly, 19,* 473–492.

Leadbeater, B. J., Blatt, S. J., & Quinlan, D. M. (1995). Gender-linked vulnerabilities to depressive symptoms, stress, and problem behaviors in adolescents. *Journal of Research on Adolescence, 5,* 1–29.

Lewinsohn, P. M., Clarke, G. N., Seeley, J. R., & Rohde, P. (1994). Major depression in community adolescents: Age at onset, episode duration, and time to recurrence. *Journal of the American Academy of Child & Adolescent Psychiatry, 33,* 809–818.

Lyubomirsky, S., Caldwell, N. D., & Nolen-Hoeksema, S. (1998). Effects of ruminative and distracting responses to depressed mood on retrieval of autobiographical memories. *Journal of Personality and Social Psychology, 75,* 166–177.

Lyubomirsky, S., & Nolen-Hoeksema, S. (1995). Effects of self-focused rumination on negative thinking and interpersonal problem solving. *Journal of Personality and Social Psychology, 69,* 176–190.

Maartens, L. W. F., Knottnerus, J. A., & Pop, V. J. (2002). Menopausal transition and increased depressive symptomatology: A community based prospective study. *Maturitas, 42,* 195–200.

Maccoby, E. E., & Jacklin, C. N. (1974). *The psychology of sex differences.* Stanford, CA: Stanford University Press.

Maciejewski, P. K., & Mazure, C. M. (in press). Fear of criticism and rejection mediates an association between childhood emotional abuse and adult onset of depression. *Cognitive Therapy and Research.*

Maciejewski, P. K., Prigerson, H. G., & Mazure, C. M. (2001). Sex differences in event-related risk for major depression. *Psychological Medicine, 31,* 593–604.

Mazure, C. M. (1998). Life stressors as risk factors in depression. *Clinical Psychology: Science and Practice, 5,* 291–313.

Mazure, C. M., Bruce, M. L., Maciejewski, P. K., & Jacobs, S. C. (2000). Adverse life events and cognitive-personality characteristics in the prediction of major depression and antidepressant response. *American Journal of Psychiatry, 157,* 896–903.

Miranda, J., & Persons, J. B. (1988). Dysfunctional attitudes are mood-state dependent. *Journal of Abnormal Psychology, 97,* 76–79.

Nazroo, J. Y., Edwards, A. C., & Brown, G. W. (1997). Gender differences in the onset of depression following a shared life event: A study of couples. *Psychological Medicine, 27*, 9–19.

Newcomb, M. D., Huba, G. J., & Bentler, P. M. (1981). A multidimensional assessment of stressful life events among adolescents: Derivation and correlates. *Journal of Health and Social Behavior, 22*, 400–415.

Nolen-Hoeksema, S. (1990). *Sex differences in depression*. Stanford, CA: Stanford University Press.

Nolen-Hoeksema, S. (1998, August). *Contributors to the gender difference in rumination*. Paper presented at the 106th Annual Convention of the American Psychological Association, San Francisco.

Nolen-Hoeksema, S. (2002). Gender differences in depression. In I. H. Gotlib & C. L. Hammen (Eds.), *Handbook of depression* (pp. 492–509). New York: Guilford Press.

Nolen-Hoeksema, S. (2004). The response styles theory. In C. Papageorgiou & A. Wells (Eds.), *Depressive rumination: Nature, theory, and treatment* (pp. 107–124). New York: Wiley.

Nolen-Hoeksema, S., & Davis, C. G. (1999). "Thanks for sharing that": Ruminators and their social support networks. *Journal of Personality and Social Psychology, 77*, 801–814.

Nolen-Hoeksema, S., & Girgus, J. S. (1994). The emergence of gender differences in depression in adolescence. *Psychological Bulletin, 115*, 424–443.

Nolen-Hoeksema, S., & Jackson, B. (2001). Mediators of the gender difference in rumination. *Psychology of Women Quarterly, 25*, 37–47.

Nolen-Hoeksema, S., & Larson, J. (1999). *Coping with loss*. Mahwah, NJ: Erlbaum.

Nolen-Hoeksema, S., Larson, J., & Grayson, C. (1999). Explaining the gender difference in depression. *Journal of Personality and Social Psychology, 77*, 1061–1072.

Oddone-Paolucci, E., Genius, M. L., & Violato, C. (2001). A meta-analysis of the published research on the effects of child sexual abuse. *Journal of Psychology, 135*, 17–36.

Paykel, E. S., Myers, J. K., Dienelt, M. N., Klerman, G. L., Lindenthal, J. J., & Pepper, M. P. (1969). Life events and depression: A controlled study. *Archives of General Psychiatry, 21*, 753–760.

Pearlin, L., & Johnson, J. (1977). Marital status, life-strains and depression. *American Sociological Review, 42*, 704–715.

Perris, H. (1984). Life events and depression, Part 1: Effect of sex, age, and civil status. *Journal of Affective Disorders, 7*, 11–24.

Peterson, C., & Seligman, M. E. (1984). Causal explanations as a risk factor for depression: Theory and evidence. *Psychological Review, 91*, 347–374.

Reynolds, K. A., Helgeson, V. S., Selgman, H., Janicki, D., Page-Gould, E., & Wardle, M. (in press). Impact of interpersonal conflict on individuals high on unmitigated communion. *Journal of Applied Social Psychology*.

Rose, D. T., & Abramson, L. Y. (1992). Developmental predictors of depressive cognitive style: Research and theory. In D. Cicchetti & S. L. Toth (Eds.), *Rochester symposium on developmental psychopathology: Vol. IV* (pp. 323–349). Hillsdale, NJ: Erlbaum.

Ruddy, N., & McDaniel, S. (1995). Domestic violence in primary care: The psychologist's role. *Journal of Clinical Psychology in Medical Settings, 2,* 46–69.

Russell, D. E. H. (1984). *Sexual exploitation.* Beverly Hills, CA: Sage.

Rutter, M., Silberg, J., O'Connor, T., & Simonoff, E. (1999). Genetics and child psychiatry II. Empirical research findings. *Journal of Child Psychology and Psychiatry, 40,* 19–55.

Salber, P. R., & McCaw, B. (2000). Barriers to screening for intimate partner violence: Time to reframe the question. *American Journal of Preventative Medicine, 19,* 276–278.

Saunders, B., Kilpatrick, D., Hanson, R., Resnick, H., & Walker, M. (1999). Prevalence, case characteristics, and long-term psychological correlates of child rape among women: A national survey. *Child Maltreatment, 4,* 187–200.

Seeman, M. V. (1997). Psychopathology in women and men: Focus on female hormones. *American Journal of Psychiatry, 154,* 1641–1647.

Shansky, R. M., Glavis-Bloom, C., Lerman, D., McRae, P., Benson, C., Miller, K., et al. (2004). Estrogen mediates sex differences in stress-induced prefrontal cortex dysfunction. *Molecular Psychiatry, 9,* 531–538.

Shors, T. J., & Leuner, B. (2003). Estrogen-mediated effects on depression and memory formation in females. *Journal of Affective Disorders, 74,* 85–96.

Shors, T. J., Pickett, J., Wood, G. E., & Paczynski, M. (1999). Acute stress enhances estrogen levels in the female rat. *Stress, 3,* 163–171.

Siegel, S. J., & Alloy, L. B. (1990). Interpersonal perceptions and consequences of depressive-significant other relationships: A naturalistic study of college roommates. *Journal of Abnormal Psychology, 99,* 361–373.

Silberg, J., Pickles, A., Rutter, M., Hewitt, J., Simonoff, E., Maes, H., et al. (1999). The influence of genetic factors and life stress on depression among adolescent girls. *Archives of General Psychiatry, 56,* 225–232.

Spence, J., Helmreich, R., & Holahan, C. (1979). Negative and positive components of psychological masculinity and femininity and their relationships to self-reports of neurotic and acting out behaviors. *Journal of Personality and Social Psychology, 37,* 1673–1682.

Steiner, M. (1992). Female-specific mood disorders. *Clinical Obstetric Gynecology, 35,* 599–611.

Steiner, M., Born, L., & Martin, P. (2000). Menarche and mood disorders in adolescence. In M. Steiner, K. Yonkers, & E. Erikkson (Eds.), *Disorders in women* (pp. 247–268). London: Martin Dunitz.

Steiner, M., & Dunn, E. (1996). The psychobiology of female-specific mood disorders. *Infertility and Reproductive Medical Clinics of North America, 7,* 297–313.

Steiner, M., Dunn, E., & Born, L. (2003). Hormones and mood: From menarche to menopause and beyond. *Journal of Affective Disorders, 74,* 67–83.

Tamres, L., Janicki, D., & Helgeson, V. S. (2002). Sex differences in coping behavior: A meta-analytic review. *Personality and Social Psychology Review, 6,* 2–30.

Teasdale, J. D. (1988). Cognitive vulnerability to persistent depression. *Cognition and Emotion, 2,* 247–274.

Teasdale, J. D., & Dent, J. (1987). Cognitive vulnerability to depression: An investigation of two hypotheses. *British Journal of Clinical Psychology, 26,* 113–126.

Tjaden, P., & Thoennes, N. (1998). *Prevalence, incidence and consequence of violence against women: Findings from the National Violence Against Women Survey. Research in brief.* Washington, DC: U.S. Department of Justice, National Institute of Justice.

Turner, R. J., & Avison, W. R. (1989). Gender and depression: Assessing exposure and vulnerability to life events in a chronically strained population. *Journal of Nervous and Mental Disease, 177,* 433–455.

Twenge, J., & Nolen-Hoeksema, S. (2002). Age, gender, race, SES, and birth cohort differences on the Children's Depression Inventory: A meta-analysis. *Journal of Abnormal Psychology, 111,* 578–588.

Uhlenhuth, E. H., & Paykel, E. S. (1973). Symptom intensity and life events. *Archives of General Psychiatry, 28,* 473–477.

U.S. Census Bureau. (2004). *Evidence from Census 2000 about earnings by detailed occupation for men and women.* Retrieved June 25, 2004, from http://www.census.gov

U.S. Department of Health and Human Services. (2001). *Mental health: Culture, race, and ethnicity: A supplement to mental health: A report of the Surgeon General.* Rockville, MD: U.S. Department of Health and Human Services, Public Health Service, Office of the Surgeon General.

Wagner, B. M., & Compas, B. E. (1990). Gender, instrumentality and expressivity: Moderators of the relation between stress and psychological symptoms during adolescence. *American Journal of Community Psychology, 18,* 383–406.

Ward, A., Lyubomirsky, S., Sousa, L., & Nolen-Hoeksema, S. (2003). Can't quite commit: Rumination and uncertainty. *Personality and Social Psychology Bulletin, 29,* 96–107.

Weiss, J. M. (1991). Stress-induced depression: Critical neurochemical and electrophysiological changes. In J. I. Madden (Ed.), *Neurobiology of learning, emotion, and affect* (pp. 123–154). New York: Raven Press.

Weiss, E. L., Longhurst, J. G., & Mazure, C. M. (1999). Childhood sexual abuse as a risk factor for depression in women: Psychosocial and neurobiological correlates. *American Journal of Psychiatry, 156,* 816–828.

Widom, C. S. (1999). Posttraumatic stress disorder in abused and neglected children grown up. *American Journal of Psychiatry, 156,* 1223–1229.

Wood, G., & Shors, T. J. (1998). Stress facilitates classical conditioning in males but impairs conditioning in females through activational influences of ovarian hormones. *Proceedings of the National Academy of Sciences, 95,* 4066–4071.

Young, E., & Korszun, A. (1999). Women, stress, and depression: Sex differences in hypothalamic–pituitary–adrenal axis regulation. In E. Leibenluft (Ed.), *Gender differences in mood and anxiety disorders: From bench to bedside* (pp. 31–52). Washington, DC: American Psychiatric Press.

Young, E. A., Midgley, A. R., Carlson, N. W., & Brown, M. B. (2000). Alteration in the hypothalamic–pituitary–ovarian axis in depressed women. *Archives of General Psychiatry, 57,* 1157–1162.

Zahn-Waxler, C. (2000). The development of empathy, guilt, and internalization of distress: Implications for gender differences in internalizing and externalizing problems. In R. Davidson (Ed.), *Wisconsin symposium on emotion: Vol. 1. Anxiety, depression, and emotion* (pp. 222–265). Oxford, England: Oxford University Press.

Zubenko, G. S., Hughes, H. B., Maher, B. S., Stiffler, J. S., Zubenko, W. N., & Marazita, M. L. (2002a). Genetic linkage of region containing the *CREB1* gene depressive disorders in women from families with recurrent, early-onset major depression. *American Journal of Medical Genetics, 114,* 980–987.

Zubenko, G. S., Hughes, H. B., Stiffler, J. S., Zubenko, W. N., & Kaplan, B. B. (2002b). Genome survey for susceptibility loci for recurrent, early-onset major depression: Results at 10cM resolution. *American Journal of Medical Genetics, 114,* 413–422.

Treatment and Prevention of Depression in Women

Rajita Sinha and A. John Rush

D epression is now recognized as a chronic disorder marked by relapses over time and, as noted in chapter 1 (this volume), women are about twice as likely as men to suffer an initial episode of depression and, thus, more likely to require effective episode treatment and prevention. The good news is that efficacious pharmacological and behavioral treatments for depression are available, and there is clear evidence for effective maintenance therapies to reduce or prevent recurrent depression

Preparation of this chapter was supported, in part, by National Institutes of Health Grants K12-DA14038 and P50-DA09241.

As with other chapters in this volume, this integrative review draws heavily on the contributions of all of the participants of the American Psychological Association Summit 2000 on Women and Depression but especially focuses on the contributions of the following manuscripts: "Pharmacotherapy of Depression in Women" by Kimberly Yonkers; "Hormones and Depression in Women" by Patricia Kroboth; "Psychotherapy for Women With Depression" by Steven Hollon; "Alternative Treatments for Depression: The Quest for Empirical Support" by Rachel Manber; "Preventing Depression in Women" by Ricardo Muñoz; "Sex Difference in Depressed Substance Abusers" by Rajita Sinha and Bruce Rounsaville; "Personality and Depression in Women: Implications for Treatment" by Thomas Widiger; and "Lesbians and Depression: Emerging Issues in Research on Morbidity, Treatment, and Prevention" by Susan Cochran.

(Depression Guideline Panel, 1993; Frank et al., 1990; Frank, Kupfer, Wagner, McEachran, & Cornes, 1991; Greden, 2001; Rush & Kupfer, 2001).

However, despite the knowledge that depression is chronic and relapsing and that treatment can be effective, a relatively small percentage of women with major depression seek or are referred for treatment of depression. Recent evidence on the use of mental health services indicates that only 22% of those with major depressive disorder are adequately treated for their illness (Kessler et al., 2003), and that the number of women who are either untreated or inadequately treated for depression is higher than those who seek specialized treatment for depression (Kessler et al., 1994). These estimates suggest a tremendous need for the further development of treatment and prevention strategies, particularly for periods of high risk in women, and they point to the importance of understanding that depression is a serious public health problem. This chapter reviews the available empirically tested treatments and prevention approaches, seeks to generate a perspective on what research is needed in this area going forward, and argues for the value of implementing empirically based treatments.

Pharmacological Treatment of Depression in Women

Several early studies and more recent data have shown that there are gender differences in the efficacy of antidepressant agents. As reviewed by Yonkers and Brawman-Mintzer (2002), Raskin (1974) documented early evidence that gender moderates response to antidepressant agents. In a study examining the effects of imipramine, chlorpromazine, phenelzine, and diazepam versus placebo, imipramine was no better than placebo for young women, although it was efficacious for men and older women. In contrast, the monoamine oxidase inhibitor (MAOI) phenelzine was more effective than placebo in young women. Other studies have reported this somewhat weaker response to tricyclic antidepressants (TCAs; e.g., imipramine) in younger women. Hamilton (1995) conducted a meta-analysis of published imipramine trials that presented outcomes by subject gender and showed that 62% of men, but only 51% of women ($p < .001$), were considered imipramine responders.

A more recent large multisite study compared the selective serotonin reuptake inhibitor (SSRI) sertraline with the TCA imipramine for the treatment of chronic depression and found that women were more likely to respond to sertraline than to imipramine, whereas men were more likely to respond favorably to imipramine than to sertraline (Kornstein et al., 2000). Furthermore, researchers also found a differential gender response to sertraline compared with imipramine for chronic mild depressive disorders (Yonkers, Clark, & Trivedi, 1997). Yonkers and Brawman-Mintzer (2002) reported that women had a 20% higher rate of response to an SSRI as compared with men (64% in women and 42% in men, $p < .02$). There is also some evidence, however, that the response to fluoxetine as compared with TCA is equivalent in women (Lewis-Hall, Wilson, Tepner, & Koke, 1997). A recent study (Quitkin et al., 2002) examined a large data set to determine gender differences in antidepressant response and included responses of patients treated with TCAs, MAOIs, fluoxetine, and placebo. Findings indicated that men and women had equivalent responses to TCAs and fluoxetine, whereas women responded better than did men to MAOIs. These data, combined with the Kornstein et al. (2000) study, point to gender-specific differences in types of antidepressants, with effects of MAOIs and sertraline showing significant gender differences in treatment response, although the data are more mixed when it comes to gender differences in effects of TCAs and fluoxetine. Although fluoxetine and sertraline are both SSRIs, there are metabolic differences in these drugs as well as differences in the extent of their effects on serotonin and catecholamine systems, which could account for their differential effects on men and women (Yonkers & Brawman-Mintzer, 2002). For example, several investigators found gender differences in the metabolism of sertraline (Ronfeld, Tremaine, & Wilner, 1997; Warrington, 1991). Though this result may be related to the differential response among men and women found by some, plasma levels are not typically associated with response so other explanations require exploration.

Some evidence suggests that women differentially absorb, distribute, and metabolize antidepressant medications, and that the gender-specific environment—gender-specific hormones or variation in receptor densities—may account for pharmacotherapeutic differences between men and women (Kroboth, 2000). New research suggests that changing the balance between gender-specific hormones across the reproductive life cycle of women can significantly affect the functioning of various neurotransmitter systems. For example, research has indicated that older women who take hormone replacement therapy (HRT) respond better to SSRIs for depression as compared with women not taking HRT (Liu et al., 2004; Schneider et al., 1997). Recent evidence also supports the efficacy of estradiol treatment for depressive disorders in endocrinologically confirmed perimenopausal women (Soares, Almeida, Joffe, & Cohen, 2001). Although estrogen's antidepressant effects are less clear in postmenopausal women, greater evidence for efficacy exists among perimenopausal women (Cohen et al., 2003; Morrison et al., 2004).

The research cited here indicates gender differences in response to sertraline, TCAs, and MAOIs. Well-controlled treatment studies suggest that gonadal steroids have significant effects on negative mood symptoms at specific periods during the reproductive life cycle while also altering the biochemical milieu such that they change the therapeutic response to antidepressants. Other somatic approaches to the treatment of depression still need to be examined in terms of gender-specific response. These include electroconvulsive therapy (ECT), a longstanding treatment, as well as emerging new treatments using brain and nerve stimulation such as repetitive Transcranial Magnetic Stimulation (rTMS; see Burt, Bisanby, & Sackheim, 2002; O'Reardon, Blummer, Peshek, Pradilla, & Pimiento, 2005) and vagus nerve stimulation (VNS; see Nahas et al., 2005) for initial and maintenance therapy.

Psychosocial Treatment of Depression in Women

In contrast to the gender differences in the pharmacological efficacy of medications for the treatment of depression, there are few demonstrated gender differences in response to psychosocial treatments for depression (Hollon, 2000). Hollon suggested several possible reasons why known gender differences are few. First, because studies were not designed to examine gender difference, and the majority of individuals enrolled in psychosocial treatment research studies of depression have been women. Thus, psychosocial treatment outcome data obtained thus far are applicable to depression in women and can be implemented in this group but do not address gender differences. Second, gender differences in rates of depression may reflect the likelihood of becoming depressed, but once depression has occurred, the mechanisms underlying affective distress and remediation could be similar for men and women. Finally, therapists may treat women and men differently in psychosocial treatments, as empirically validated psychosocial treatments do allow for sufficient internal flexibility, permitting therapists to adjust the nature of the interventions to accommodate the needs of women and men. Although more research with balanced numbers of women and men in psychosocial treatment outcome studies is needed, clear psychosocial treatment findings are ready for implementation in women with depression.

Evidence suggests the efficacy of cognitive–behavioral therapy (CBT) and interpersonal therapy (IPT) for the treatment of depression in women, whereas dynamic therapies of depression have not fared as well in efficacy studies, partly because of the lack of standardization of these therapies. As reviewed by Hollon (2000), IPT is as effective as antidepressants in the reduction of acute distress in women and in forestalling relapse and recurrence in non-treatment-resistant, depressed outpatients. There is also evidence that IPT may have delayed effects on the social functioning and the quality of relationships in women that build over time. One of the few indications of gender differences is that men appear to respond more rapidly than do women to the combination of IPT and a TCA, whereas IPT without a TCA is an effective treatment for women with depression (Frank, Carpenter, & Kupfer, 1988).

In reviewing studies of the efficacy of CBT for depression, Hollon (2000) concluded that CBT is effective in the treatment of depression in women, although there is some evidence that it may not be as effective for women with severe depression. Nonetheless, the findings to date are consistent with the notion that CBT has an enduring effect that continues to protect against relapse and recurrence after treatment completion, with evidence suggesting that keeping women in treatment can do the same.

Though researchers have not studied behavioral treatments such as skills training, self-control training, problem-solving therapy, and contingency management as extensively as they have studied IPT or CBT, they have found these approaches to be superior to minimal treatment and as effective as other established treatments such as antidepressant medications (Jarrett & Rush, 1994). In addition, although studies report some efficacy for behavioral marital therapy and for marital and family therapy, this finding needs further examination (Clarkin et al., 1990; Jacobson, Dobson, Fruzzetti, Schmaling, & Salusky, 1991). Finally, recent studies of the cognitive–behavioral analytic system of psychotherapy indicate evidence for the preferential effectiveness of a combination of pharmacotherapy and psychosocial treatments in complex and chronic depression, and for the combination in chronically depressed outpatients (Keller et al., 2000; Ninan et al., 2002).

As depression is a chronic relapsing disorder, research has been conducted to determine effective treatments for prevention of relapse. Substantial data indicate that psychosocial therapies, such as IPT and CBT, show positive effects as maintenance therapies by addressing residual symptoms of depression and reducing the recurrence of depressive episodes (Fava, Grandi, Zielezny, Canestari, & Morphy, 1994; Fava, Grandi, Zielezny, Rafanelli, & Canestrari, 1996; Frank et al., 1990; Jarrett et al., 1998, 2001; Paykel et al., 1999). These treatments alone, and in combination with medications, as continuation phase treatments or in preventing relapse have shown positive outcomes. In addition, newer approaches, such as mindfulness-based cognitive therapy, that include some alternative interventions, such as yoga and mindfulness meditation, have shown benefit in reducing relapse in women with recurrent depressive episodes (Segal, Williams, & Teasdale, 2002; Teasdale, 1999). These findings support the implementation of CBT, IPT, and mindfulness-based cognitive therapy as maintenance phase therapies that target prevention of recurrent episodes and relapse.

Thus, although gender differences in response to psychosocial treatments for depression are few, substantial evidence supports the implementation of these treatments both for reducing acute distress and, just as important, for preventing recurrence and relapse of future episodes. Key aspects of implementation include providing access to and covering the cost of these efficacious treatments. Adequate health coverage for the full dose of psychosocial treatment necessary to ensure a positive treatment response is one health care delivery issue that needs to be addressed.

Alternative Therapies for Depression

The popularity of alternative forms of treatment for relief of depression has surged. These treatments include herbal medicine, acupuncture, bright light, sleep deprivation, exercise, and stress management. These alternatives are popular because antidepressant medications are not universally effective or universally acceptable to all clients and patients. Manber and colleagues (2002) reported that over 30% of individuals completing medication research protocols are nonresponsive to active treatments, and that 50% of individuals with chronic depression are nonresponders. Furthermore, 25% or more of participants may prematurely terminate treatment because of medication adverse effects or other undetermined reasons (Keller et al., 2000). Though psychosocial treatments are efficacious, they remain inaccessible and unaffordable for many patients. It is not surprising, then, that depression is among the most common conditions for which patients seek alternative, in place of conventional, therapies (Eisenberg et al., 1998). Thus, there is a need to investigate and examine the efficacy of alternative approaches.

Manber et al. (2002) systematically reviewed and summarized current research findings on alternative therapies. This review indicates that some unconventional treatments hold promise as alternative or complementary treatments for depression and have the potential to contribute to its long-term management. Exercise and stress reduction methods, particularly yoga, appear to have support as adjuncts to conventional treatments. Research has found that exercise improves mood; some evidence, although limited, also suggests that it can lead to remission of major depression, particularly in older adults (Blumenthal et al., 1999;

North, McCullagh, & Tran, 1990). Among the stress reduction therapies, yoga and mindfulness meditation appear to show benefit in individuals with dysthymia (Janakiramaiah et al., 1998) and in preventing relapse among individuals with a history of chronic recurrent depression (Segal et al., 2002; Teasdale et al., 2000).

Manber et al. (2002) discussed the promise of acupuncture as an alternative treatment for major depression. Several studies, but only a few randomized, controlled trials, suggested that acupuncture treatment is effective in reducing depressive symptoms in depressed women (Allen, Schnyer, & Hitt, 1998; Gallagher, Allen, Hitt, Schnyer, & Manber, 2001). An important aspect of its effectiveness is that it is well-tolerated, with 13% dropout rates. Whereas this initial evidence supports its use as an alternative treatment for major depression, larger studies are under way to further evaluate its efficacy, particularly during pregnancy and lactation periods.

Several studies have also assessed St. John's wort, which was found to be superior to placebo and comparable to standard TCAs in some studies (Linde et al., 1996). More recent studies have found St. John's wort comparable in efficacy to imipramine and to SSRIs (Harrer et al., 2000; Phillip, Kohnen, & Hiller, 1999). However, a recent multicenter trial in the United States found that St. John's wort was not more efficacious than placebo in the treatment of major depressive disorders (Hypericum Depression Trial Study Group, 2002), but neither was sertraline in this study.

Manber et al. (2002) also concluded that though bright light exposure is effective for seasonal affective disorder, it is significantly less effective for the treatment of nonseasonal major depression. In addition, on the basis of current evidence, sleep deprivation is unlikely to become a useful alternative therapy for depression.

Prevention of Depression in Women

As rates of depression in women are double that in men and such gender differences in onset of major depression become evident in adolescence, Le, Muñoz, Ippen, and Stoddard (2003) poignantly made the case for targeting prevention of depression in young women. They pointed out that (a) clinical depression is related to many other health problems such as smoking, substance abuse, and heart disease in women; (b) women who develop major depression during pregnancy are more likely to have recurrent episodes during the next 5 years and beyond; and (c) the children of depressed mothers are more likely to develop cognitive, social, and mood problems. These facts highlight the need and rationale for implementation of early intervention and prevention findings and for providing specific recommendations for future research in this area. As the first episode of depression generally sets in motion a chronic course, a primary goal is to prevent the first episode. To address the highest risk areas, Le and colleagues suggested that preventive efforts focus on adolescent girls, women at risk for smoking and other substance abuse, and women about to become mothers. Furthermore, they emphasized that prevention efforts in these groups of women should focus on those most at risk for depressive symptoms and least likely to use traditional mental health services, such as low-income or minority women.

Findings on prevention efforts in adolescents indicate that 12- and 16-session group interventions focusing on cognitive and behavioral factors, such as cognitive or social problem-solving skills and adaptive coping strategies, significantly lower the risk of developing major depression compared with control groups (Clarke et al., 1995, 2001; Gillham, Reivich, Jaycox, & Seligman, 1995; Jaycox, Reivich, Gillham, & Seligman, 1994). School-based prevention efforts targeting middle and high school children are feasible and often relatively easy to implement (Rice & Meyer, 1994). However, data on gender differences in this area are also limited, and studies examining the efficacy of prevention interventions should report effects by gender (Gillham, Shatté, & Freres, 2000). Also limited are studies of prevention efforts for ethnic minority girls.

Researchers have examined some prevention efforts for women at risk for smoking and women about to become mothers. Le et al. (2003) cited evidence supporting the use of mood management interventions for smokers at risk for developing depression and those with histories of depression, as these groups are at high risk of developing recurrent depression. They are also at high risk for failure to quit smoking. Studies show management strategies that target mood regulation in addition to smoking cessation yield significantly higher quit rates than do interventions without such mood-oriented strategies (Hall, Muñoz, & Reus, 1994; Hall et al., 1998; Muñoz, Marin, Posner, & Perez-Stable, 1997).

Le et al. (2003) similarly made the case for prevention of major depression during pregnancy and postpartum. Psychological interventions that target depression prevention for these high-risk groups are emerging. Olds and colleagues (Olds et al., 1998a, 1998b) conducted several studies that evaluated the effect of prenatal and early childhood home-visitation programs by public health nurses among low-income African American and European American women, following them for 15 years after their child's birth. Findings indicated improved health-related behaviors, decreased criminal behaviors and reduced substance abuse, and improved infant caregiving abilities, but no improvement in depression scores. In an ongoing project, Le and colleagues (2003) are conducting a 12-week course during pregnancy and four booster sessions during the first postpartum year on depression prevention. The course teaches mood management skills embedded in materials related to pregnancy and parenting. Results from this study are still forthcoming.

More research is needed to establish the indications for and efficacy of prevention efforts; as a consequence, data to inform widespread prevention efforts are limited, especially in the prevention of the first episode in adolescents where the need for efficacy is clear.

Factors Affecting the Risk of Developing Depression and Treatment Outcome

Sinha and Rounsaville (2002) indicated that substance abuse can be both a vulnerability factor in the development of depression and a risk factor for treatment failure and recurrence of depression. Substance use disorders are known to be more common among depressed young women than among healthy control young women (Rao, Daley, & Hammen, 2000). Thus, effective treatment strategies to address such comorbidity are imperative in the treatment of depression in women. When depression is the primary diagnosis and substance abuse is secondary, treatment of depression concurrent with substance abuse is crucial to reduce the likelihood of recurrence of depression and substance abuse. In such cases, after achieving initial abstinence (i.e., detoxification or postacute withdrawal) from the primary drug of abuse, research has shown that treatment of underlying depression is of benefit in preventing relapse (Cornelius et al., 1997). Furthermore, addition of mood management strategies to standard cognitive–behavioral treatment of substance abuse improves both depression and substance use outcomes (Brown, Evans, Miller, Burgess, & Mueller, 1997; Hall, Muñoz, & Reus, 1994; Hall et al., 1998). However, researchers have not specifically examined gender effects, and future studies need to assess whether these findings hold true in both men and women with comorbid substance abuse and depression. Because depression is often substance-induced and depressive symptomatology is a common feature of the acute and protracted withdrawal states associated with nicotine, alcohol, opiates, and cocaine, diagnosing depression in individuals with comorbid substance abuse and depression can be challenging. Nonetheless, evidence suggests that depressive symptoms in substance-abusing patients can improve with antidepressant medication, despite the modest effects of this approach on improving substance use outcomes (Kosten, Markou, & Koob, 1998; Nunes et al., 1998; Stein et al., 2004). These data indicate that the treatment of depressive symptoms that can contribute to substance relapse is an important treatment target in comorbid depression and substance use disorders.

Another factor known to affect risk of developing depression and risk of recurrence in women is the presence of personality disorders. Widiger and Anderson (2003) reviewed the research on personality factors, particularly presence of neuroticism and dependent personality disorder, as a vulnerability factor for developing mood disorders and for recurrence of these disorders. The key finding relevant for implementation is the significant association between these personality traits and vulnerability for mood disorders. In light of this association, assessment of personality factors is needed, particularly after improvement in a depressive episode. The continuing presence of maladaptive behaviors would suggest the need for treatment of personality disorders.

Dialectical behavior therapy (DBT; Koerner & Linehan, 2000; Linehan, 1993) has shown initial promise in the treatment of borderline personality disorders. Health plans are growing interested in paying for this treatment because of evidence that it reduces the use of expensive services. Whether DBT also reduces the likelihood of recurrence of future depressive episodes is not known. Nonetheless, clinical assessment of personality factors during treatment and remission from depressive episodes will allow for comprehensive approaches to treatment and, thus, could reduce the likelihood of future episodes of depression in women.

Cochran (2001) discussed the influence of sexual orientation on the risk of developing psychiatric and substance use disorders. She cited several well-controlled prospective studies indicating that homosexuality appears to function as a risk factor for psychiatric disorders, particularly depression and substance use disorders (Cochran, 2001; Cochran & Mays, 2000b; Sandfort, de Graaf, Bijl, & Schnabel, 2001). Furthermore, the risk appears to be greatest during adolescence and young adulthood, and it declines as individuals age (Cochran & Mays, 2000a; Sorenson & Roberts, 1997). Although elevated risk is now increasingly well-documented, reasons for the increased risk are unclear. Cochran (2001) discussed evidence to support the role of social stigma as a risk factor for psychological distress, particularly depression, anxiety symptoms, and substance use (Dohrenwend, 2000; Kessler, Mickelson, & Williams, 1999).

Finally, citing evidence that lesbians and gay men are higher consumers of treatment services than are heterosexual women and men, Cochran (2001) addressed treatment effectiveness for depression problems among lesbians and gay men. She raised the question of whether treatments in homosexual groups are equally effective as treatments in heterosexual depressed individuals, and whether standard care addresses the problems of depressed lesbians and gay men. She pointed out that though recent studies show that mental health providers do not view homosexuality as pathological, they still frequently evidence both attitudinal and behavioral responses to sexual minority clients that may not be conducive to positive outcomes (Bieschke, McClanahan, Tozer, Grzegorek, & Park, 2000; Cochran, 2001). These responses include having difficulty recalling information the patient has provided, avoiding topics that make the therapist uncomfortable, and either over- or underemphasizing the relevance of sexual orientation in the client's problems. From an implementation point of view, at a minimum, providers need to address their own attitudes and biases toward sexual orientation and become sensitive to addressing the problems of this population in treatment.

Recommendations for Research and Practice

1. Prevent the first episode of depression in women. As there is strong evidence that gender differences in the onset of major depression begin in adolescence (Cyranowski, Frank, Young, & Shear, 2000), it is important to prevent the first episode of depression in women by implementing mood management training for preadolescents as part of health and hygiene education in schools. Such training would, of course, require practitioners to provide preteens themselves with greater education and awareness about the increased risk of depression with onset of puberty in girls, and involve the school staff, including the school nursing, counseling, and teaching staff. Furthermore, improved dissemination of the signs and symptoms of mood and behavioral changes that accompany increased negative affect in preteen and teen years would be beneficial. Given the considerable ongoing education on various aspects of health, biology, sex education, and substance use in schools, educational systems may easily integrate specific skills training on mood management and added awareness of mental illness. The integration of such information and training into the school systems not only will educate the adolescents and school staff but also will increase awareness and provide information and education to parents.

In addition to mood management training in school and in individual treatment plans, increased public education on (a) the link between mood changes and risk of depression, (b) behavioral signs and symptoms of depressive onset in children, (c) management of early signs and symptoms in preteen and adolescent girls, and (d) the short- and long-term effects of depression on life functioning, via widespread public service announcements, information bulletin boards at schools, community centers, and the Internet, is warranted. Educators may model these efforts along the lines of recent efforts to reduce drug use in children. Such efforts have shown some markers of positive outcomes as evidenced by the increased awareness of drug effects among children, parents, and educators.

2. *Widely implement empirically based treatments for depression in women.* Practitioners can avail themselves of training in empirically validated treatments for depression. In addition, professional support is needed in the effort to influence the health insurance industry to cover the cost and increase the accessibility of psychosocial treatments. Practitioners and their professional societies can be influential in ensuring that psychosocial treatments with established efficacy, such as IPT and CBT, are supported for the number of sessions required to produce positive outcomes. Coverage of less than the adequate number of sessions would be parallel to covering pharmacological treatments at inadequate doses to produce benefit, an effect that is not beneficial from either a cost or a treatment delivery perspective.

In addition to providing full reimbursement for evidence-based psychosocial treatments, it is imperative that treatments are available in different languages with adaptation to diverse cultures, and for access and implementation in minority populations. Thus, the translation and adaptation of psychosocial treatment manuals into Spanish and the major Asian languages may be of benefit, especially in increasing access for low-income, minority women who are known to be less likely to seek treatment for depression. Along a similar vein, provision of ongoing education and supervision in these treatments for providers who are directly delivering care to these populations would be important. Both providers and consumers can benefit from greater knowledge of the effective dosing and frequency of contact for psychosocial treatments. This education can, of course, be done within the format of continuing education and medical education credits, peer-group consultation that provides a forum for colleagues to discuss clinical issues pertaining to treatment, and public service dissemination strategies discussed in an earlier section.

In contrast to psychosocial treatments, pharmacological treatments are widely used and covered by most health plans. Women's documented response to sertraline and to MAOIs needs to be considered by practitioners when they evaluate patients for pharmacotherapy. In addition, in light of gender differences in pharmacokinetics of antidepressant medications, health care plans should cover the cost of testing blood levels of selected medications (e.g., TCAs) where this has been shown to be clinically useful. This testing is particularly important in those individuals with high side-effect profiles, in nonresponders, or in those with concurrent general medical conditions. Furthermore, consumer education on the effective amount, dose, and frequency of medications would be particularly important in ensuring the appropriate use of antidepressant medications.

Finally, practitioners should be encouraged to assess comorbid factors that affect treatment outcome because these factors may be addressed by specialized treatments. Active substance abuse can seriously reduce the effectiveness of treatment of depression. Thus, evaluation of the extent of substance use and treatment of substance abuse by referral to specialized treatment services or provision of integrated treatment, such as CBT with mood management, is a useful strategy in the management of such comorbidity. In a similar manner, the effect of personality factors and sexual orientation, which may significantly affect onset, course, and treatment outcome of depressive illness, should be evaluated carefully. This evaluation may be especially useful with reference to sexual orientation, as matching patients to providers who are sensitive to the needs of the homosexual population would be particularly useful in improving treatment outcomes.

3. Prevent relapse of depressive episodes with maintenance therapies. The third area of recommendation focuses on prevention of relapse and recurrence of depressive episodes. Depression is likely best viewed through a sustained disease management treatment approach because increased rates of recurrence lead to a more chronic course of the illness with reduced effectiveness of standard treatments. Providers need to consider the implementation of psychosocial therapies, such as IPT and cognitive therapies including CBT and mindfulness-based cognitive therapy, as maintenance therapies to reduce residual symptoms of depression and recurrence of depressive episodes. These treatments alone and in combination with medication as continuation phase treatments are effective in preventing recurrent relapse in women with depression and can be implemented effectively with a chronic disease management approach to depression.

4. *Support gender-specific treatment research.* Research on the treatment of depression in women is needed in several areas. Early research has documented gender differences in treatment response to antidepressants. However, the underlying factors associated with these differences are poorly understood. Yonkers and Brawman-Mintzer (2002) maintained that the differences may likely be associated with gender differences in the pharmacokinetics and pharmacodynamics of antidepressants. Evidence suggests that gonadal steroids, such as estrogen, may have direct antidepressant effects while also altering the biochemical milieu such that these hormones change the therapeutic response to antidepressants. Future research on the interaction between hormones, depressive symptomatology, and treatment responses would be particularly useful in developing targeted gender-specific treatments for depression in women.

Future research is also needed on the role of gender in treating the comorbidity of depression with personality disorders and with substance use disorders. As indicated in the previous sections, presence of these illnesses both increases the risk of major depression, especially in women, and increases the likelihood of treatment failure and recurrence of depressive episodes. In the majority of depression treatment trials, comorbid conditions have been an exclusion criterion, so there is little information on how to treat women with such comorbidity effectively. With high rates of comorbidity and greater cost burden due to recurrence in these comorbid groups, it is imperative to develop and evaluate treatments for depression comorbid with personality disorders and with substance use disorders in women. To maximize efforts, researchers should focus on how interventions need to differ for women and men. Further evaluation of the effectiveness of cognitive–behavioral treatments for substance use disorders and for borderline personality disorder (e.g., DBT) in women with comorbid depression (Carroll, 1998; Koerner & Linehan, 2000; Linehan, 1993) is needed. Mood management strategies added to standard cognitive–behavioral treatments for substance use disorders have seen some success in individuals with histories of depression (Brown et al., 1997; Hall et al., 1996, 1998), but future studies need to evaluate gender-specific effects.

5. *Investigate mechanisms for increasing access to care.* With data suggesting that only 22% of women with major depression obtain adequate treatment for depression, it is clear that one of the major challenges in dealing with depression is increasing access to mental health services. Thus, there is a need for developing and evaluating effective treatment engagement strategies for women with depression, especially low-income and minority women who are less likely to have access to mental health care because of social and familial barriers. Development and evaluation of treatments for pregnant and lactating women and those with refractory depression is also necessary to provide empirically valid treatments for women with these conditions. Finally, data indicate that lesbians and gay men are higher consumers of services than are nonhomosexual groups (Cochran, 2001). Thus, research that evaluates whether specialized treatments, such as affirmative therapies (Bieschke et al., 2000), enhance treatment outcomes in these populations can go a long way in improving treatment for this population and reducing costs associated with services to lesbians and gay men.

6. *Support research on the efficacy of prevention interventions in women.* Though research on etiology and treatment is necessary to understand the underlying causes of depression and to treat depression in women once it has developed, effective prevention strategies must be developed to help prevent depression. Le et al. (2003) outlined several key areas of future prevention research to curb the rise in rates of depression in adolescent girls and adult women. There is a need to identify subgroups of women who are at high and imminent risk for major depression. Though it is well-known that preteen and teenage girls are at high risk, women who are smokers and those who are pregnant and

lactating are in high-risk subgroups as well, and it is important to systematically assess this risk in other subgroups, such as minority and low-income women and single mothers. Furthermore, studies of adolescents could benefit from long-term follow-up to assess whether preventing depression in adolescence protects women from developing depression later in the life cycle.

Researchers have documented the impact that major depression in women has on other serious social and physical health problems (Murray & Lopez, 1996). However, the proportion of physical and mental health problems in women attributable to depression needs to be clarified as does the effect of treating and preventing depression on the risk of other conditions and disorders, such as smoking, substance abuse, and cardiovascular disease. Thus, future intervention studies should address multiple outcomes, including healthy physical development and prevention of psychopathology. Explicit assessment of collateral public health problems, such as smoking, other substance abuse, unplanned pregnancies, marital problems, school performance, job performance, and physical health, in prevention studies will result in more comprehensive findings on depression prevention. Subject recruitment in research protocols should include those who are at high risk, including low-income and minority women, as well as those who are non-English-speaking. Recruitment of these groups of women would require research collaborations with community settings such as school systems, primary care clinics, and religious and community networks. Including a representative sample of women in prevention and treatment research studies will ultimately lead to the development of interventions that are easily generalizable, with widespread data on response to empirically valid interventions in all subgroups of women.

Recommendations for Policy With Regard to Treatment and Prevention

1. Develop and implement a widespread public education campaign. The Global Burden of Disease Study reported that by the year 2020, depression will be second only to ischemic heart disease in current patterns of mortality and disability (Murray & Lopez, 1996). These data require classification of major depression in women as a major public health problem, which necessitates widespread coordinated attention in public education, early detection and intervention, and relapse prevention. Information on the gender-specific nature of depression, including significantly higher rates in women, differential risk and protective factors, and early signs and symptoms, and effective treatment options needs to be widely disseminated to the public. Indeed, once policymakers acknowledge depression as a serious public health problem in women, there will be a greater impetus and commitment toward such coordinated public outreach efforts. Widespread education initiatives will increase awareness, reduce stigma, and allow for greater access to prevention and treatment opportunities.

2. *Use a chronic disease management model in approaching depression.* It would be prudent for health care delivery systems to approach depression with the chronic disease management model that requires support for its initial prevention, episode treatment, and prevention of recurrence. Such efforts would be similar to those required by chronic illnesses such as hypertension, congestive heart failure, asthma, and diabetes. The chronic disease framework would emphasize the importance of prevention and early detection efforts, particularly via provision of gender-specific public health service messages, dissemination of information on its nature, causes, and effective treatments, and sponsorship of empirically validated prevention programs to reduce risk of developing depression in specific targeted subgroups of girls and women. It would also provide a basis for provision of early detection information and encourage the use of evidence-based pharmacological, psychosocial, and alternative treatments to consumers and health care delivery providers. Finally, the chronic disease model will necessitate the provision of critical information on recurrence and relapses and effective treatment alternatives to prevent relapse.

3. *Focus efforts on parity for mental health services.* It is crucial that health care policymakers address the current disparity that exists between mental and physical health coverage. It is well-known that depression in women increases the risk of onset and worsens the outcomes of other general medical disorders, such

as congestive heart failure, hypertension, and substance use disorders (Depression Guideline Panel, 1993). Providing parity between mental health care financing and physical health care financing will improve outcomes and reduce the burden of both physical and mental illnesses in women.

References

Allen, J. J. B., Schnyer, R. N., & Hitt, S. K. (1998). The efficacy of acupuncture in the treatment of major depression in women. *Psychological Science, 9,* 397–401.

Bieschke, K. J., McClanahan, M., Tozer, E., Grzegorek, J. L., & Park, J. (2000). Programmatic research on the treatment of lesbian, gay, and bisexual clients: The past, present, and the course for the future. In R. M. Perez, K. A. DeBord, & K. J. Bieschke (Eds.), *Handbook of counseling and psychotherapy with lesbian, gay, and bisexual clients* (pp. 309–336). Washington, DC: American Psychological Association.

Blumenthal, J. A., Babyak, M. A., Moore, K. A., Craighead, W. E., Herman, S., Khatri, P. R., et al. (1999). Effects of exercise training on older patients with major depression. *Archives of Internal Medicine, 159,* 2349–2356.

Brown, R. A., Evans, D. M., Miller, I. W., Burgess, E. S., & Mueller, T. I. (1997). Cognitive–behavioral treatment for depression in alcoholism. *Journal of Consulting and Clinical Psychology, 65,* 715–726.

Burt, T., Lisanby, S. H., & Sackheim, H. A. (2002). Neuropsychiatric applications of transcranial magnetic stimulation: A meta-analysis. *International Journal of Neuropsychopharmacology, 5,* 73–103.

Carroll, K. M. (Ed.). (1998). *A cognitive–behavioral approach: Treating cocaine addiction* (NIH Publication No. 98-4308). Rockville, MD: National Institute on Drug Abuse.

Clarke, G. N., Hawkins, W., Murphy, M., Sheeber, L., Lewinsohn, P. M., & Seeley, J. R. (1995). Targeted prevention of unipolar depressive disorder in an at-risk sample of high school adolescents: A randomized trial of a group cognitive intervention. *Journal of the American Academy of Child & Adolescent Psychiatry, 34,* 312–321.

Clarke, G. N., Hornbrook, M., Lynch, F., Polen, M., Gale, J., Beardslee, W., et al. (2001). A randomized trial of a group cognitive intervention for preventing depression in adolescent offspring of depressed parents. *Archives of General Psychiatry, 58,* 1127–1134.

Clarkin, J. F., Glick, I. D., Haas, G. L., Spencer, J. H., Lewis, A., Peyser, J., et al. (1990). A randomized clinical trial of inpatient family intervention: V. Results for affective disorders. *Journal of Affective Disorders, 18,* 17–28.

Cochran, S. D. (2001). Emerging issues in research on lesbians' and gay men's mental health: Does sexual orientation really matter? *American Psychologist, 56,* 931–947.

Cochran, S. D., & Mays, V. M. (2000a). Lifetime prevalence of suicidal symptoms and affective disorders among men reporting same-sex sexual partners: Results from the NHANES III. *American Journal of Public Health, 90,* 573–578.

Cochran, S. D., & Mays, V. M. (2000b). Relation between psychiatric syndromes and behaviorally defined sexual orientation in a sample of the U.S. population. *American Journal of Epidemiology, 151,* 516–523.

Cohen, L. S., Soares, C. N., Poitras, J. R., Prouty, J., Alexander, A. B., & Shifren, J. L. (2003). Short-term use of estradiol for depression in perimenopausal and postmenopausal women: A preliminary report. *American Journal of Psychiatry, 160,* 1519–1522.

Cornelius, J. R., Salloum, I. M., Ehler, J. G., Jarrett, P. J., Cornelius, M. D., Perel, J. M., et al. (1997). Fluoxetine in depressed alcoholics: A double-blind, placebo-controlled trial. *Archives of General Psychiatry, 54,* 700–705.

Cyranowski, J. M., Frank, E., Young, E., & Shear, M. K. (2000). Adolescent onset of the gender difference in lifetime rates of major depression: A theoretical model. *Archives of General Psychiatry, 57,* 21–27.

Depression Guideline Panel. (1993). *Depression in primary care: Vol. 2. Treatment of major depression. Clinical Practice Guideline, Number 5* (AHCPR Publication No. 93-0551). Rockville, MD: U.S. Department of Health and Human Services.

Dohrenwend, B. P. (2000). The role of adversity and stress in psychopathology: Some evidence and its implications for theory and research. *Journal of Health and Social Behavior, 41,* 1–19.

Eisenberg, D. M., Davis, R. B., Ettner, S. L., Appel, S., Wilkey, S., Van Rompay, M., & Kessler, R. C. (1998, November 11). Trends in alternative medicine use in the United States, 1990–1997: Results of a follow-up national survey. *Journal of the American Medical Association, 280,* 1569–1575.

Fava, G. A., Grandi, S., Zielezny, M., Canestari, R., & Morphy, M. A. (1994). Cognitive behavioral treatment of residual symptoms in primary major depressive disorder. *American Journal of Psychiatry, 151,* 1295–1299.

Fava, G. A., Grandi, S., Zielezny, M., Rafanelli, C., & Canestrari, R. (1996). Four-year outcome for cognitive behavioral treatment of residual symptoms in major depression. *American Journal of Psychiatry, 153,* 945–947.

Frank, E., Carpenter, L. L., & Kupfer, D. J. (1988). Sex differences in recurrent depression: Are there any that are significant? *American Journal of Psychiatry, 145,* 41–45.

Frank, E., Kupfer, D. J., Perel, J. M., Cornes, C., Jarrett, D. B., Mallinger, A. G., et al. (1990). Three-year outcomes for maintenance therapies in recurrent depression. *Archives of General Psychiatry, 47,* 1093–1099.

Frank, E., Kupfer, D. J., Wagner, E. F., McEachran, A. B., & Cornes, C. (1991). Efficacy of interpersonal psychotherapy as a maintenance treatment of recurrent depression: Contributing factors. *Archives of General Psychiatry, 48,* 1053–1059.

Gallagher, S. M., Allen, J. J., Hitt, S. K., Schnyer, R. N., & Manber, R. (2001). Six-month depression relapse rates among women treated with acupuncture. *Complementary Therapies in Medicine, 9*, 216–218.

Gillham, J. E., Reivich, K. J., Jaycox, L. H., & Seligman, M. E. P. (1995). Prevention of depressive symptoms in schoolchildren: Two-year follow-up. *Psychological Science, 6*, 343–351.

Gillham, J. E., Shatté, A. J., & Freres, D. R. (2000). Preventing depression: A review of cognitive–behavioral and family interventions. *Applied & Preventive Psychology, 9*, 63–88.

Greden, J. F. (2001). Clinical prevention of recurrent depression. The need for paradigm shifts. In J. M. Oldham (Series Ed.), & J. F. Greden (Vol. Ed.), *Review of psychiatry: Vol. 20. Treatment of recurrent depression* (pp. 143–170). Washington, DC: American Psychiatric Press.

Hall, S. M., Muñoz, R. F., & Reus, V. I. (1994). Cognitive–behavioral intervention increases abstinence rates for depressive-history smokers. *Journal of Consulting and Clinical Psychology, 62*, 141–146.

Hall, S. M., Reus, V. I., Muñoz, R. F., Sees, K. L., Humfleet, G., Hartz, D. T., et al. (1998). Nortriptyline and cognitive–behavioral therapy in the treatment of cigarette smoking. *Archives of General Psychiatry, 55*, 683–690.

Hall, S. M., Sees, K. L., Muñoz, R. F., Reus, V. I., Duncan, C., Humfleet, G. L., & Hartz, D. T. (1996). Mood management and nicotine gum in smoking treatment: A therapeutic contact and placebo-controlled study. *Journal of Consulting and Clinical Psychology, 64*, 1003–1009.

Hamilton, J. (1995). *Sex and gender as critical variables in psychotropic drug research.* Pittsburgh, PA: University of Pittsburgh Press.

Harrer, G., Schmidt, U., Kuhn, U., & Biller, A. (2000). Comparison of equivalence between the St. John's wort extract LoHyp-57 and fluoxetine. *Arneimittelforschung, 49*, 289–296.

Hollon, S. D. (2000, October). *Psychotherapy for women with depression.* Paper presented at the American Psychological Association Summit 2000 on Women and Depression, Queenstown, MD.

Hypericum Depression Trial Study Group. (2002, April 10). Effect of Hypericum perforatum (St. John's wort) in major depressive disorder: A randomized controlled trial. *Journal of the American Medical Association, 287*, 1807–1814.

Jacobson, N. S., Dobson, K., Fruzzetti, A. E., Schmaling, K. B., & Salusky, S. (1991). Marital therapy as a treatment for depression. *Journal of Consulting and Clinical Psychology, 59*, 547–557.

Janakiramaiah, N., Gangadhar, B. N., Murthy, P. J. N. V., Harish, M. G., Shetty, T. K., Subbakrishna, D. K., et al. (1998). Therapeutic efficacy of Sudarshan Kriya Yoga (SKY) in dysthymic disorder. *NIMHANS Journal, 16*, 21–28.

Jarrett, R. B., Basco, M. R., Risser, R., Ramanan, J., Marwill, M., Kraft, D., & Rush, A. J. (1998). Is there a role for continuation phase cognitive therapy for depressed outpatients? *Journal of Consulting and Clinical Psychology, 66*, 1036–1040.

Jarrett, R. B., Kraft, D., Doyle, J., Foster, B. M., Eaves, G. G., & Silver, P. C. (2001). Preventing recurrent depression using cognitive therapy with and without a continuation phase: A randomized clinical trial. *Archives of General Psychiatry, 58,* 381–388.

Jarrett, R. B., & Rush, A. J. (1994). Short-term psychotherapy of depressive disorders: Current status and future directions. *Psychiatry, 57,* 115–132.

Jaycox, L. H., Reivich, K. J., Gillham, J., & Seligman, M. E. P. (1994). Prevention of depressive symptoms in school children. *Behaviour Research and Therapy, 32,* 801–816.

Keller, M. B., McCullough, J. P., Klein, D. N., Arnow, B., Dunner, D. L., Gelenberg, A. J., et al. (2000). A comparison of nefazodone, the cognitive behavioral analysis system of psychotherapy, and their combination for the treatment of chronic depression. *New England Journal of Medicine, 342,* 1462–1470.

Kessler, R. C., Berglund, P., Demler, O., Jin, R., Koretz, D., Merikangas, K. R., et al. (2003, June 18). The epidemiology of major depressive disorder: Results from the National Comorbidity Survey Replication (NCS–R). *Journal of the American Medical Association, 289,* 3095–3105.

Kessler, R. C., McGonagle, K. A., Zhao, S., Nelson, C. B., Hughes, M., Eshleman, S., et al. (1994). Lifetime and 12-month prevalence of *DSM–III–R* psychiatric disorders in the United States: Results from the National Comorbidity Survey. *Archives of General Psychiatry, 51,* 8–19.

Kessler, R. C., Mickelson, K. D., & Williams, D. R. (1999). The prevalence, distribution, and mental health correlates of perceived discrimination in the United States. *Journal of Health and Social Behavior, 40,* 208–230.

Koerner, K., & Linehan, M. M. (2000). Research on dialectical behavior therapy for patients with borderline personality disorder. *Psychiatric Clinics of North America, 23,* 151–167.

Kornstein, S. G., Schatzberg, A. F., Thase, M. E., Yonkers, K. A., McCulough, J. P., Keitner, G. I., et al. (2000). Gender differences in treatment response to sertraline versus imipramine in chronic depression. *American Journal of Psychiatry, 157,* 1445–1452.

Kosten, T. R., Markou, A., & Koob, G. F. (1998). Depression and stimulant dependence: Neurobiology and pharmacotherapy. *Journal of Nervous and Mental Disease, 186,* 737–745.

Kroboth, P. D. (2000, October). *Hormones and depression in women.* Paper presented at the American Psychological Association Summit 2000 on Women and Depression, Queenstown, MD.

Le, H., Muñoz, R. F., Ippen, C. G., & Stoddard, J. L. (2003, September 15). Treatment is not enough: We must prevent major depression in women. *Prevention & Treatment, 6*(2), 1–43.

Lewis-Hall, F. C., Wilson, M. G., Tepner, R. G., & Koke, S. C. (1997). Fluoxetine versus tricyclic antidepressants in women with major depressive disorder. *Journal of Women's Health, 6,* 337–343.

Linde, K., Ramirez, G., Mulrow, C. D., Pauls, A., Weidenhammer, W., & Melchart, D. (1996). St. John's wort for depression—An overview and meta-analysis of randomised clinical trials. *British Medical Journal, 313*, 253–258.

Linehan, M. M. (1993). *Cognitive–behavioral treatment of borderline personality disorder.* New York: Guilford Press.

Liu, P., He, F. F., Bai, W. P., Yu, Q., Shi, W., Wu, Y. Y., et al. (2004). Menopausal depression: Comparison of hormone replacement therapy and hormone replacement therapy plus fluoxetine. *Chinese Medical Journal, 117*, 189–194.

Manber, R., Allen, J., & Morris, M. (2002). Alternative treatments for depression: Empirical support and relevance to women. *Journal of Clinical Psychiatry, 63*, 628–640.

Morrison, M. F., Kallan, M. J., Ten Have, T., Katz, I., Tweedy, K., & Battistini, M. (2004). Lack of efficacy of estradiol for depression in postmenopausal women: A randomized, controlled trial. *Biological Psychiatry, 55*, 406–412.

Muñoz, R. F., Marin, B. V., Posner, S. F., & Perez-Stable, E. J. (1997). Mood management mail intervention increases abstinence rates for Spanish-speaking Latino smokers. *American Journal of Community Psychology, 25*, 325–343.

Murray, C. J., & Lopez, A. D. (1996, November 1). Evidence-based health policy: Lessons from the Global Burden of Disease Study. *Science, 274*, 740–743.

Nahas, Z., Marangell, L. B., Husain, M. M., Rush, A. J., Sackheim, H. A., Lisanby, S. H., et al. (2005). Two-year outcome of vagus nerve stimulation (VNS) for treatment of major depressive episodes. *Journal of Clinical Psychiatry, 99*, 1097–1104.

Ninan, P. T., Rush, A. J., Crits-Christoph, P., Kornstein, S. G., Manber, R., Thase, M. E., et al. (2002). Symptomatic and syndromal anxiety in chronic forms of major depression: Effect of nefazadone, cognitive behavioral analysis system of psychotherapy, and their combination. *Journal of Clinical Psychiatry, 63*, 434–441.

North, T. C., McCullagh, P., & Tran, Z. V. (1990). Effect of exercise on depression. *Exercise and Sport Sciences Reviews, 18*, 379–415.

Nunes, E. V., Quitkin, F. M., Donovan, S. J., Deliyannides, D., Ocepek-Welikson, K., Koenig, T., & Brady, R. (1998). Imipramine treatment of opiate-dependent patients with depressive disorders. *Archives of General Psychiatry, 55*, 153–160.

Olds, D., Henderson, C. J., Kitzman, H., Eckenrode, J., Cole, R., & Tatelbaum, R. (1998a). The promise of home visitation: Results of two randomized trials. *Journal of Community Psychology, 26*, 5–21.

Olds, D., Pettitt, L. M., Robinson, J., Henderson, C. J., Eckenrode, J., Kitzman, H., et al. (1998b). Reducing risks for antisocial behavior with a program of prenatal and early childhood home visitation. *Journal of Community Psychology, 26*, 65–83.

O'Reardon, J. P., Blummer, K. H., Peshek, A. D., Pradilla, R. R., & Pimiento, P. C. (2005). Long-term maintenance for major depressive disorder with rTMS. *Journal of Clinical Psychiatry, 66,* 1524–1528.

Paykel, E. S., Scott, J., Teasdale, J. D., Johnson, A. L., Garland, A., Moore, R., et al. (1999). Prevention of relapse in residual depression by cognitive therapy: A controlled trial. *Archives of General Psychiatry, 56,* 826–835.

Phillip, M., Kohnen, R., & Hiller, K. O. (1999). Hypericum extract versus imipramine or placebo in patients with moderate depression: Randomized multicenter study of treatment for eight weeks. *British Medical Journal, 319,* 1534–1539.

Quitkin, F. M., Stewart, J. W., McGrath, P. J., Taylor, B. P., Tisminetzky, M. S., Petkova, E., et al. (2002). Are there differences between women's and men's antidepressant responses? *American Journal of Psychiatry, 159,* 1848–1854.

Rao, U., Daley, S. E., & Hammen, C. (2000). Relationship between depression and substance use disorders in adolescent women during the transition to adulthood. *Journal of the American Academy of Child & Adolescent Psychiatry, 33,* 215–222.

Raskin, A. (1974). Age-sex differences in response to antidepressant drugs. *Journal of Nervous and Mental Disease, 159,* 120–130.

Rice, K. G., & Meyer, A. L. (1994). Preventing depression among young adolescents: Preliminary process results of a psycho-educational intervention program. *Journal of Counseling & Development, 73,* 145–152.

Ronfeld, R. A., Tremaine, L. M., & Wilner, K. D. (1997). Pharmacokinetics of sertraline and its N-demethyl metabolite in elderly and young male and female volunteers. *Clinical Pharmacokinetics, 32,* 22–30.

Rush, J., & Kupfer, D. (2001). Strategies and tactics in the treatment of depression. In G. O. Gabbard (Ed.), *Treatments of psychiatric disorders: Vol. 2. Section 6* (3rd ed., pp. 1417–1439). Washington, DC: American Psychiatric Press.

Sandfort, T. G. M., de Graaf, R., Bijl, R. V., & Schnabel, P. (2001). Same-sex sexual behavior and psychiatric disorders: Findings from the Netherlands Mental Health Survey and Incidence Study (NEMESIS). *Archives of General Psychiatry, 58,* 85–91.

Schneider, L. S., Small, G. W., Hamilton, S. H., Bystritsky, A., Nemeroff, C. B., & Meyers, B. S. (1997). Estrogen replacement and response to fluoxetine in a multicenter geriatric depression trial: Fluoxetine collaborative study group. *American Journal of Geriatic Psychiatry, 5,* 97–106.

Segal, Z. V., Williams, J. M. G., & Teasdale, J. D. (2002). *Mindfulness-based cognitive therapy for depression: A new approach to preventing relapse.* New York: Guilford Press.

Sinha, R., & Rounsaville, B. J. (2002). Sex differences in depressed substance abusers. *Journal of Clinical Psychiatry, 63,* 616–627.

Soares, C. N., Almeida, O. P., Joffe, H., & Cohen, L. S. (2001). Efficacy of estradiol for the treatment of depressive disorders in perimenopausal women: A double-blind, randomized, placebo-controlled trial. *Archives of General Psychiatry, 58,* 529–534.

Sorenson, L., & Roberts, S. J. (1997). Lesbians' uses of and satisfaction with mental health services: Results from Boston Lesbian Health Project. *Journal of Homosexuality, 33,* 35–49.

Stein, M. D., Solomon, D. A., Herman, D. S., Anthony, J. L., Ramsey, S. E., Anderson, B. J., & Miller, I. W. (2004). Pharmacotherapy plus psychotherapy for treatment of depression in active injection drug users. *Archives of General Psychiatry, 61,* 152–159.

Teasdale, J. D. (1999). Emotional processing, three modes of mind, and the prevention of relapse in depression. *Behaviour Research and Therapy, 37*(Suppl. 1), 53–57.

Teasdale, J. D., Segal, Z. V., Williams, J. M. G., Ridgeway, V. A., Soulsby, J. M., & Lau, M. A. (2000). Prevention of relapse/recurrence in major depression by mindfulness-based cognitive therapy. *Journal of Consulting and Clinical Psychology, 68,* 615–623.

Warrington, S. J. (1991). Clinical implications of the pharmacology of sertraline. *International Clinical Psychopharmacology, 6,* 11–21.

Widiger, T. A., & Anderson, K. G. (2003). Personality and depression in women. *Journal of Affective Disorders, 74,* 59–66.

Yonkers, K. A., & Brawman-Mintzer, O. (2002). The pharmacological treatment of depression: Is gender a critical factor? *Journal of Clinical Psychiatry, 63,* 610–615.

Yonkers, K. A., Clark, R. H., & Trivedi, M. H. (1997). The psychopharmacological treatment of nonmajor mood disorders. In A. J. Rush (Ed.), *Systematic medication management: Modern problems of pharmacopsychiatry* (pp. 146–166). Basel, Switzerland: Karger.

3

Targeting Populations of Women for Prevention and Treatment of Depression

Jill M. Cyranowski and Ellen Frank

A lthough women as a group are at heightened risk for depression, a variety of biological, psychosocial, and demographic factors may place certain groups of women at higher risk than others. Women do not experience the psychological turmoil of depression in a vacuum, but within the rich context of their individual lives. Special considerations may, therefore, be indicated for the development and implementation of effective yet practical interventions for targeted populations of women.

The particular focus of this chapter is depression as it may occur in the context of reproductive events experienced by

Preparation of this chapter was supported, in part, by National Institute of Mental Health Grants MH49115, MH30915, and MH64144.

As with other chapters in this volume, this integrative review draws heavily on the contributions of all of the participants of the American Psychological Association Summit 2000 on Women and Depression, but especially focuses on the contributions of the following manuscripts: "Depression During the Menopausal Transition" by Nancy Avis; "Aging Women and Depression" by Margaret Gatz and Amy Fiske; "Chronic Depression in Women" by Susan Kornstein; "What Research Suggests for Depressed Women With Children" by Myrna M. Weissman and Peter Jensen; "Depression During Pregnancy and the Postpartum Period" by Katherine L. Wisner, James Perel, Kathleen Peindl, and Barbara Gracious; and "Premenstrual Disorders: Bridging Research With Clinical Reality" by Kimberly Yonkers, Teri Pearlstein, and Robert Rosenheck.

women, including menarche, pregnancy and postpartum, and the menopausal transition. These reproductive events occur within the context of women's interpersonal and professional lives, and may interact with social or developmental life challenges associated with adolescence and young adulthood, midlife, and late life. The rewards and challenges of multiple caregiving roles typically held by women, which may include caregiving for children, spouses or partners, aging parents, and extended social networks, exist throughout these developmental phases. These caregiving demands exist, for most women, in addition to their ever-growing presence in the paid workforce. The extent and importance of women's caregiving roles, moreover, highlight the ease with which the negative consequences of depression may spread across women's social networks, adversely affecting their children, partners, families, friends, and communities.

The past 20 years of research have underscored the chronic, recurrent, and seriously undertreated nature of unipolar depressive disorder. Yet, just as no two women are alike, neither are any two depressive episodes. Depressive episodes may vary widely in symptom profile, intensity, and course. Episodes may occur independently or in conjunction with coexisting physical or psychiatric problems. Thus, the varying faces of this disorder warrant consideration with regard to risk profiles and targeted intervention strategies.

The targeted populations of women with depression covered in this chapter are neither comprehensive nor exhaustive, but do focus on critical junctures in the lives of women. It is clear that there are many groups of women who are at particular risk of depression, who may require special intervention considerations and whose needs go unmet by current mental health policy and service organizations.

Adolescence

As shown by accumulating evidence in developmental psychopathology, the gender gap in adult depression traces back to a dramatic shift in lifetime prevalence rates that occurs sometime between the ages of 10 and 15 (Angold & Rutter, 1992; Kessler, McGonagle, Swartz, Blazer, & Nelson, 1993). Although absolute rates of depression continue to rise for both men and women throughout adulthood, the relative predominance of depression in women that begins with puberty essentially does not change for the next 35 to 40 years, roughly paralleling women's reproductive years (Kessler et al., 1993; Weissman, Bruce, Leaf, Florio, & Holzer, 1991). In fact, it has been argued that "the period between ages 10 and 15 appears to be critical for understanding why females are more likely to experience depression than males" (Frank & Young, 2000).

As a consequence, adolescence represents an important target for research programs designed to understand the mechanisms underlying the gender difference in lifetime depression rates. The adolescent transition also represents a unique opportunity for primary interventions designed to educate preadolescents and their care providers (including parents, peers, teachers, coaches, school nurses, and pediatricians) about depression, as well as secondary intervention programs designed to prevent depression onset among at-risk populations.

Reproductive Status Events of Adolescence: Menarche

Major transitions in both biological and psychosocial spheres mark the adolescent years. Dramatic changes in circulating hormone levels occur throughout late childhood and early adolescence. Developmental changes in the endocrine system include adrenarche, or the onset of sex steroid secretion by the adrenal glands that begins between the ages of 6 and 8 years, and gonadarche, or the maturation of the gonads beginning at age 9 or 10. In light of gonadarche's concurrence with the onset of the gender difference in depression, research has implicated pubertal changes in circulating gonadal hormones as exerting direct or potentiating effects on the central nervous system that relate to mood disturbances in adolescent women.

Changes in gonadal hormones are also associated with profound morphological changes during puberty, such as the emergence of secondary sex characteristics including increased body hair (especially pubic), breast development, and related body changes. Some have argued that the sexes experience pubertal changes in physical appearance quite differently, with males viewing growth and body development as positive, and females experiencing menarche, breast development, and increased levels of body fat as negative—particularly if the timing of these changes occurs prior to that found in their peer group (see Stattin & Magnusson, 1990).

Brooks-Gunn and Warren (1989) suggested that the "turning on" of the endocrine system at puberty may explain increases in negative affect among adolescent females. In one study, these researchers found that self-reported negative affect increased in 10- to 14-year-old females during pubertal estrogen rise. It is notable, however, that estrogen levels accounted for only 4% of the variance in negative affect. In contrast, the combination of negative life events and the interaction of negative life events with estrogen change accounted for 17% of the variance in self-reported depressed mood (Brooks-Gunn & Warren, 1989).

Social and Developmental Roles During Adolescence: Adolescent Transitions and Gender Role Socialization

In addition to the biological and physical changes associated with puberty, adolescents undergo significant transitions in social roles. Adolescent developmental transitions include major changes in school environments as well as significant changes experienced across parental and peer relationships. For many, adolescence also brings the initiation and intensification of romantic and sexual relationships.

By adolescence, females are more likely than males to have experienced certain negative life events, such as sexual abuse (Cutler & Nolen-Hoeksema, 1991). Research has established the role of psychosocial factors and negative life events in depression onset and recurrence in the adult literature. Indeed, considerable evidence suggests that negative life events and chronic psychosocial problems place individuals in general, and females in particular, at risk for major depressive episodes (Brown & Harris, 1978; Lewinsohn, Hoberman, & Rosenbaum, 1988; Maciejewski, Prigerson, & Mazure, 2001; Paykel et al., 1969; see also chap. 1, this volume). Recent data, moreover, suggest that pubertal maturation may sensitize females to the depressogenic effects of negative life events (Angold, Worthman, & Costello, 1997; Ge, Lorenz, Conger, Elder, & Simons, 1994), and, particularly, those events with negative interpersonal consequences (Cyranowski, Frank, Young, & Shear, 2000).

Females tend to display a strong affiliative style in their social relationships. This tendency toward affiliation in females, and the preference for close emotional communication and intimacy within interpersonal relationships (Bakan, 1966; Baker-Miller, 1986; Feingold, 1994) has been attributed to biological factors as well as gender role socialization. Although gender differences in affiliative style are apparent well before adolescence (Maccoby, 1990), social pressures to conform to stereotypically feminine versus masculine roles may intensify during the pubertal transition. This process, referred to as *gender intensification,* has received empirical support. For example, Larson and Richards (1989, 1991) found that as girls progress through adolescence, they spend less time alone and more time engaged in social activities with peers. Adolescent girls also spend more time talking than do their male peers and, with increasing age, their conversations reflect an increasing interpersonal focus (Raffaelli & Duckett, 1989).

The process of female gender-role socialization may prepare adolescent females for the caregiving roles they may assume during subsequent developmental stages, such as caring for young children in early adulthood, aging parents in midlife, and ailing spouses or partners in late life. At the same time, however, researchers have theorized that this pubertal intensification in affiliative orientation may sensitize postpubertal females to the depressogenic effects of negative life events, and, particularly, events that represent conflicts, breaches, or losses within interpersonal relationships (see Cyranowski et al., 2000).

Early Adulthood

Although adolescence may see the emergence of the gender difference in lifetime depression rates, depression becomes most prevalent during early adulthood. Depression typically has its onset during the second and third decades of life (Burke, Burke,

Rae, & Regier, 1991). Because, for many women, this heightened risk for depression falls squarely on the childbearing and child-rearing years of early adulthood, we now focus on the implications of this demographic with regard to the safe treatment of women during pregnancy and postpartum, as well as the long-term physical, emotional, and behavioral health of young children of mothers who struggle with depression.

Reproductive Events of Early Adulthood: Pregnancy and Postpartum

Women of childbearing age are, on average, at heightened risk of experiencing depressive episodes. Approximately 9% of pregnant women and 13% of postpartum women experience major depressive disorder (MDD; O'Hara, Neunaber, & Zekoski, 1984). In women with previous episodes of postpartum depression, the risk of depressive recurrence during postpartum increases to 25% (Wisner, Gelenberg, Leonard, Zarin, & Frank, 1999; Wisner, Parry, & Piontek, 2002). Researchers believe rapid fluctuations in reproductive hormones experienced during pregnancy and postpartum contribute to the development of mood disorders in susceptible women. Nevertheless, studies have also associated stressful life events with increased risk of depression during pregnancy and postpartum (as during other times in women's lives; see Swendsen & Mazure, 2000). In light of the practical, financial, and emotional demands many women face as they manage work, childcare, and extended social demands, research should not overlook the role of life stress experienced by women during pregnancy and the postpartum period.

With regard to pregnancy and the postpartum period, the need to consider both the effects of depression and the treatment risks for the mother and the developing fetus or newborn child adds a layer of complexity to treatment decisions in this target population. For example, though healthcare providers must consider the potential adverse effects of antidepressant medications on the development of the fetus or breast-feeding infant, they also must consider fully the potential effects of untreated maternal depression on the development of the fetus or young child (Wisner et al., 2000).

The biological dysregulation of MDD, including the neuroendocrine dysfunction of the hypothalamic–pituitary–adrenal stress axis, may represent a toxic environment for the developing fetus (Wisner et al., 2000). Numerous animal studies implicate maternal stress in such adverse outcomes as fetal hypoxia, low birth weight, miscarriage, and fetal hypotension (Istvan, 1986). Practitioners must also consider the behavioral ramifications of MDD, including suicidality, social withdrawal, poor prenatal care seeking, sleep disturbance, weight loss, and substance abuse—all of which may further jeopardize the health of the mother and the development of the fetus. Finally, depression experienced during the postpartum period may undermine the mother's ability to provide developmentally appropriate infant care, reducing reciprocal mother–infant interactions and diverting attention from the infant's developmental needs. These outcomes may then result in children of depressed mothers showing an increased risk of emotional and behavioral problems (see Weissman & Jensen, 2002).

Treatment options for depression during pregnancy and postpartum include psychotherapy, antidepressant medication therapy, and electroconvulsive therapy, as well as lesser studied alternative treatments such as bright light therapy (e.g., see Epperson et al., 2004; Oren et al., 2002). These treatments are reviewed in chapter 2 (this volume).

Interpersonal psychotherapy (IPT), an empirically supported psychotherapeutic treatment for MDD, has recently been adapted to treat women with depression both during pregnancy (Spinelli, 1997) and the postpartum period (O'Hara, Stuart, Gorman, & Wenzel, 2000). Also, a group intervention based on interpersonal psychotherapy was found to be effective in preventing postpartum depression onset in a sample of at-risk, disadvantaged women (Zlotnick, Johnson, Miller, Pearlstein, & Howard, 2001). The focus of IPT on interpersonal concerns and, in particular, on interpersonal role transitions may be particularly suited to meet the needs of depressed women who recently have become mothers. Other empirically supported psychotherapies for depression may be similarly effective during pregnancy and postpartum. For example, Appleby, Warner, Whitton, and Faragher (1997) found cognitive–behavioral therapy (CBT) as well as fluoxetine to be effective for depression during the postpartum period. When available, efficacious psychotherapeutic interventions may represent a particularly attractive treatment option for those patients with serious concerns regarding the potential effects of pharmacologic treatments during pregnancy and breast-feeding.

Four recent prospective studies (Chambers, Johnson, Dick, Felix, & Jones, 1996; Kulin et al., 1998; Nulman et al., 1997; Pastuszak et al., 1993) and a critical review (Wisner et al., 1999) of relevant human and animal data examined the teratogenic effects of antidepressant medications used during pregnancy. Existing studies provide no evidence to implicate tricyclic antidepressants or SSRIs during pregnancy as causes of major birth defects or intrauterine fetal death. One study (Chambers et al., 1996) did find lower birth weights in fetuses exposed to fluoxetine after 25 weeks gestation, although growth deficits were not obtained in two other studies (Kulin et al., 1998; Nulman et al., 1997). Because of the long half-life of fluoxetine and neonates' difficulty in metabolizing this medication, Wisner and Perel (1988) have suggested strategies to taper the drug prior to delivery to minimize fetal drug load at birth.

Wisner et al. (2002) reviewed reports published on neonatal exposure to antidepressant medications during breast-feeding. The SSRI sertraline has recently been recommended as a first-line pharmacologic treatment for breast-feeding mothers, on the basis of current evidence that this agent may be used with little risk (Altshuler et al., 2001). The decision to combine breast-feeding and antidepressant therapy, however, must be made on a case-by-case basis, weighing the benefits of breast-feeding, the benefits of available treatment options, the potential risks of untreated maternal depression, and the potential and unknown risks of neonatal exposure to specific antidepressants or their metabolites.

Depressed Women With Children

The fact that peak risks for depression occur throughout women's childbearing and childrearing years has implications for the treatment of depressed women during pregnancy and postpartum, and for the physical, emotional, and behavioral health of the offspring under their care. Highlighting the prevalence of maternal depression, Weissman and colleagues have reported heightened levels of depression among mothers in various clinic samples. In one study of mothers bringing their children for psychiatric treatment, 14% screened positive for current MDD, 59% screened positive for subsyndromal depression, and 22% reported suicidal ideation or intent (Ferro, Verdeli, Pierre, & Weissman, 2000). In a study conducted in a primary care setting, 25% of mothers with children age 6 through 17 reported current depression, and 19.5% reported other psychiatric disorders (Olfson et al., 2000). As compared with mothers with other psychiatric disorders or normal controls, mothers with depression were more likely to report that their children had serious emotional problems for which they were not receiving treatment, and that they had poor relationships with their children (Weissman et al., 2004).

As reviewed by Weissman and Jensen (2002), numerous studies support a link between maternal depression and an increased risk of psychiatric disorders in offspring. For example, in one longitudinal study (Warner, Weissman, Fendrich, Wickramaratne, & Moreau, 1992; Weissman, Warner, Wickramaratne, Moreau, & Olfson, 1997), offspring of depressed parents were (a) at higher risk for onset of MDD and anxiety disorders during childhood, (b) at higher risk for MDD during adolescence, and (c) at higher risk for alcohol dependence in adolescence and early adulthood. Thus, the negative impact of depression in mothers extends well beyond the emotional, behavioral, and financial functioning of the women themselves to affect the offspring under their care. Yet, as noted by Weissman and Jensen (2002), estimates of the economic cost of depression have ignored projections of the impact of this disorder on the offspring of affected individuals, including the increased rates of both medical and psychiatric problems found in these at-risk samples. Finally, the psychiatric risks of familial depression appear to be transmitted not only to children, but also to grandchildren (Warner, Weissman, Mufson, & Wickramaratne, 1999).

Midlife and Late-Life Populations

For some women, midlife may include a worsening of premenstrual mood symptoms, or premenstrual dysphoric disorder (PMDD). The onset of premenstrual complaints typically occurs during early adulthood, and a number of young adults experience severe forms of this disorder. However, because these symptoms tend to worsen with age until relieved by the onset of menopause, this section includes a review of these disorders. A second reproductive status event of midlife is the menopausal transition. Although it was previously believed that rates of MDD in the general population increased in women following menopause, the evidence reviewed in the following section questions this notion.

A variety of social and interpersonal stressors may accompany developmental transitions of midlife and late life. For example, as young adults increasingly delay the onset of childbirth, some women find themselves sandwiched between competing caregiving demands of children and aging parents. As women progress to late life, caregiving demands may include physically or cognitively disabled spouses or partners. More often than not, women must balance these multiple caregiving demands with the demands of full-time employment and associated occupational stressors. In late life, women may also face increasing health problems and functional decrements, financial stressors, and bereavement-related issues.

Reproductive Status Events of Midlife

Premenstrual disorders. Women may experience an array of premenstrual mood symptoms across the age range. Although the onset of these complaints typically occurs during early adulthood, women commonly report that their symptoms worsen with age (Johnson, McChesney, & Bean, 1988). Thus, the prevalence of severe premenstrual mood disorders appears to be higher in midlife populations (Campbell, 1976; Johnson et al., 1988).

Yonkers, Pearlstein, and Rosenheck (2003) categorized premenstrual complaints in ascending order of severity, ranging from minor and minimally distressing premenstrual symptoms, to the more severe and distressing premenstrual syndrome (PMS), and, finally, to PMDD as codified by the *Diagnostic and Statistical Manual of Mental Disorders* (4th ed., *DSM–IV*; American Psychiatric Association, 1994). The *DSM–IV* section of criteria sets for further study defines PMDD as including mood or anxiety complaints (such as depressed mood, mood swings, anxiety, anger, or irritability) as well as a range of associated symptoms such as decreased interest, difficulty concentrating, anergia, changes in sleep or appetite, and related physical symptoms (e.g., bloating, headaches, breast tenderness). Differentiating PMDD from other forms of PMS are the following required criteria: mood or anxiety complaints, the presence of five or more of the above-mentioned symptoms, functional impairment resulting from premenstrual complaints, and evidence that the disorder is not merely an exacerbation of another disorder, such as MDD. Finally, in light of the potential bias inherent in retrospective reporting, the *DSM–IV* requires that symptom criteria for PMDD be confirmed via prospective daily monitoring of symptoms.

As reviewed by Yonkers et al. (2003), prevalence data obtained from general community and student populations suggest that though 30% to 50% of women report minor levels of premenstrual symptoms, less than 5% report more severe and disabling symptoms (Johnson et al., 1988; Logue & Moos, 1986; Rivera-Tovar & Frank, 1990; Woods, Most, & Dery, 1982). Notably, however, prevalence rates of PMDD are likely to be higher in clinic populations (Plouffe, Stewart, Craft, Maddox, & Rausch, 1993; West, 1989), and conflicting opinions regarding the prevalence of PMDD persist. Symptoms of PMS and PMDD have been reported in a variety of crosscultural populations, with irritability ranking as the most common mood symptom in a number of studies (e.g., Mao & Chang, 1985; Merikangas, Foeldenyl, & Angst, 1993). Yonkers and colleagues reviewed data from several studies indicating that even relatively low levels of premenstrual complaints may have a deleterious impact on social and interpersonal quality-of-life domains (Campbell, Peterkin, O'Grady, & Sanson-Fisher, 1997; Hylan, Sundell, & Judge, 1999). Indeed, it is not surprising that even minor mood symptoms such as increased irritability may have a negative impact on interpersonal functioning. Moreover, a small percentage of women with severe symptoms may experience significant work-related impairments (Hylan et al., 1999; Johnson et al., 1988).

A considerable number of women who meet criteria for PMDD also have a co-occurring psychiatric diagnosis. For example, in one study (Plouffe et al., 1993), 36% of women sampled from a specialty PMS clinic met criteria for a psychiatric diagnosis. These and other findings suggest the existence of a subgroup of women with a history of MDD who display a heightened sensitivity to changes in reproductive hormone levels, such as those occurring premenstrually, as well as changes that occur during postpartum or perimenopausal reproductive transitions.

A growing body of evidence supports the effectiveness of SSRI treatment for patients with PMDD. As reviewed by Yonkers et al. (2003), 16 randomized clinical trials support the effectiveness of these antidepressant agents, particularly fluoxetine and sertraline. In general, these studies indicate that SSRIs effectively treat approximately 65% of women with PMDD, as compared with a typical 25% to 30% placebo response rate in these groups.

Although a majority of these studies have investigated the continuous use of medications, recent research supports treating women with SSRIs only during the luteal phase of the menstrual cycle (e.g., see Halbreich et al., 2002; Halbreich & Smoller, 1997; Jermain, Preece, Sykes, & Sulak, 1999; Steiner, Korzekwa, Lamont, & Wilkins, 1997; Sundblad, Hedberg, & Eriksson, 1993; Wikander et al., 1998; Young, Hurt, Benedek, & Howard, 1998). It is important to note, however, that these studies excluded women with irregular menstrual cycles and required patients to closely monitor ovulation through the use of ovulation detection kits. In light of these constraints and the lack of evidence to support luteal dosing schedules in more general clinical settings, questions remain regarding the practicality and effectiveness of this treatment approach in the general population.

Menopause and depression. The belief that a majority of women become clinically depressed following menopause has extensive historic roots, and, even today, is commonly held by patients and health care providers alike. Yet, despite widespread belief in this phenomenon, the existing epidemiologic literature does not support the notion that most women suffer from MDD following menopause. How, then, did the perceived relationship between menopause and depression come into being? In her review, Avis (2003) examined a number of methodological problems in the existing literature that may foster this perception. She argued that a number of studies in this area have relied on patient- versus population-based samples, which may include multiple treatment-seeking biases that overestimate the prevalence of mood disorders in menopausal women. In addition, Avis pointed to significant inconsistencies in the definition and measurement of both menopausal status and depressive status across studies. It is clear that these methodological issues need to be addressed in future research.

As reviewed by Avis (2003), many prospective longitudinal studies have failed to find an increase in rates of MDD following menopause (see Hallstrom & Samuelsson, 1985; Holte, 1992; Kaufert, Gilbert, & Tate, 1992; Matthews et al., 1990; Woods & Mitchell, 1996; but see also Avis, Brambilla, McKinlay, & Vass, 1994; Hunter, 1990). Instead, longitudinal data indicate that the primary predictor of depression following menopause is a prior depressive history, a finding that is not surprising given the recurrent nature of this disorder (Avis et al., 1994; Hunter, 1990; Kuh, Wadsworth, & Hardy, 1997; Porter, Penney, Russell, Russell, & Templeton, 1996). In addition, a number of studies have indicated that social factors, such as fluctuating levels of life stress, may predict a greater proportion of the variance in depressive outcomes than do the hormonal changes associated with menopause (Hallstrom & Samuelsson, 1985; Hunter, 1990; Kaufert et al., 1992).

However, accumulating research evidence does suggest that women may be at greater risk of experiencing depressive symptoms during the perimenopausal transition from regular menstrual cycling to complete cessation of menses. This transition period may range from 3 to 9 years in length (McKinlay, Brambilla, & Posner, 1992) and is marked by less predictable menstrual cycles and fluctuations in gonadal hormones. One theory linking increased depressive symptoms to perimenopause posits that vasomotor symptoms (such as hot flashes) associated with fluctuating estrogen levels during perimenopause lead to chronic sleep disturbances that, in turn, lead to irritability and mood symptoms (Lauritzen, 1973; Schmidt & Rubinow, 1991; van Keep & Kelherhals, 1974). In support of this theory, Collins and Landgren (1995) found that the obtained cross-sectional association between menopause and depressive symptoms disappeared after controlling for common vasomotor symptoms of menopause. Another study examining the association between vasomotor symptoms and depression in women seeking primary care indicated that perimenopausal women with recent vasomotor symptoms were four times more likely to be depressed than were those without vasomotor symptoms, even after controlling for depression history (Joffe et al., 2002). Other studies, however, have obtained elevated reports of depressive symptoms or psychological distress during the perimenopausal transition even after controlling for relevant vasomotor symptoms (see Bromberger et al., 2001; Freeman et al., 2004).

Although depression during menopause was long believed to be caused by a reduction or deficiency in estrogen levels following menopause, recent data suggest that the increase in depressive symptoms during perimenopause may instead be related to fluctuations in gonadal hormones that occur during the perimenopausal transition (Freeman et al., 2004). Evidence also suggests that women who report a lifetime history of depression (and, particularly, depression associated with previous periods of hormonal fluctuation such as postpartum depression and PMDD) are at heightened risk of experiencing depression recurrence during the perimenopausal transition (Collins & Landgren, 1995; Dennerstein et al., 1993; Stewart & Boydell, 1993; Woods & Mitchell, 1996).

Hormone replacement therapies (HRTs) have long been believed to lead to lower depression rates during menopause. Current evidence to support a direct effect of HRT on mood is inconsistent (Holte, 1998; Palinkas & Barrett-Connor, 1992). Well-controlled clinical trials comparing HRT with placebo have generally produced inconsistent results (Holte, 1998; Pearce, Hawton, & Blake, 1995). Recent preliminary data suggest promising results for the use of transdermal estradiol in the alleviation of depression during perimenopause (Cohen et al., 2003), and the use of a combination of estrogens and SSRIs for depression during the postmenopausal period (Soares, Poitras, & Prouty, 2003; Soares, Poitras, Prouty, Alexander, et al., 2003). It is clear that such findings are in need of replication in larger randomized, double-blind clinical trials.

Women's multiple roles at midlife and late life. Women often have multiple social roles in midlife to late life, including a variety of personal roles (mother, wife or partner, daughter, sibling, grandmother), professional roles (employee, supervisor, businesswoman, mentor), political roles, and community roles. New demands and potential sources of life stress may accompany developmental changes across social roles. Indeed, recent research suggests that the effects of stress on women's depression risk may vary by age (see Mazure & Maciejewski, 2003), highlighting the need for age-specific approaches to depression assessment, prevention, and treatment.

The challenges of women's caregiving roles may change but not cease after their children reach early adulthood and move away from home. Indeed, child-care tasks of early adulthood may diminish only to be replaced, or in some cases surpassed, by multiple adult caregiving roles later in life. For the woman at midlife, these caregiving tasks may include caring for physically or cognitively impaired parents or other aging family members. During late life, adult caregiving demands may revolve around caring for ailing spouses, partners, or siblings. These caregiving demands often compete with ongoing work demands.

With the graying of the population, the demands placed on informal or familial adult caregivers will only continue to increase. And, in line with their nurturing or caregiving roles, women tend to assume primary responsibility for adult caregiving tasks. Supporting this view, national surveys of adult caregiving estimate that approximately 70% to 75% of all adult caregivers are women (National Alliance for Caregiving and the American Association of Retired Persons, 1997; Stephens & Christianson, 1986; Stone, Cafferata, & Sangl, 1987).

A growing literature indicates that the demands of adult caregiving can have a negative impact on the psychological well-being of care providers. As compared with population norms and with noncaregiving controls, adult caregivers report higher levels of depressive symptoms, clinical depression, and anxiety (for reviews, see Schulz, O'Brien, Bookwala, & Fleissner, 1995; Schulz, Visintainer, & Williamson, 1990). Moreover, as pointed out in a review by Yee and Schulz (2000), female caregivers appear to experience excess psychiatric morbidity attributable to caregiving, as compared with male caregivers and with non-caregiving community samples.

Examining the caregiving experience in terms of a stress process model, Yee and Schulz (2000) showed that women are at greater risk for psychiatric morbidity than are men at all stages of caregiving. To begin, women are more likely than men to assume the role of primary adult caregiver. In addition, female caregivers spend more time providing caregiving assistance than do male caregivers, and are more likely to perform daily hands-on caregiving tasks such as household chores and personal care. Women also tend to remain in the caregiver role longer than do men (who are more likely to relinquish caregiving responsibilities as the care recipient becomes increasingly disabled), and are less likely than men to obtain informal assistance with caregiving responsibilities. Moreover, it would appear that female caregivers are more likely than males to place the needs of care recipients ahead of their own health care behaviors. For example, female caregivers are more likely than males to report not having enough time for rest, exercise, doctor appointments, and the like (Burton, Newson, Schulz, Hirsch, & German, 1997). Finally, Yee and Schulz (2000) pointed out that in a majority of studies, female caregivers report experiencing greater levels of caregiver burden, role strain, and role stress than do male caregivers, and that female caregivers show excess psychiatric morbidity attributable to the adult caregiving experience.

Aging and depression. Epidemiological studies examining the prevalence of depression across the life span generally have not focused on late-life depression. One study, using a large random sample of the British population, reported that sex differences in the prevalence of depression are less apparent after age 55 (Bebbington et al., 1998). This finding has led some to suggest that hormonal fluctuations during reproductive years account for higher rates of depression in women during this time. However, if higher rates of depression in women were solely due to biological vulnerability, the gender ratio should be largely unaffected by psychosocial variables; nevertheless, it is affected (Bebbington et al., 1998). It is clear that both biological and behavioral mechanisms need to be considered as researchers strive to understand the developmental trajectory of the gender gap in depression.

Because of the differential longevity of women compared with men, an increasingly large proportion of the U.S. population will be composed of women aged 65 and older. Hence, as Gatz and Fiske (2003) contended, efforts to distinguish which groups of older women may be at particular risk for depression and to determine the special diagnostic and treatment considerations for these groups are of particular importance.

The accurate assessment of depressive symptoms and disorders within aging populations may itself represent a particular challenge. As reviewed by Gatz and Fiske (2003), among older adults with late-onset depression, a subset may represent a type of vascular depression associated with structural brain changes, vascular risk factors, and cognitive impairment (Alexopoulos, Meyers, Young, Campbell, et al., 1997; Alexopoulos, Meyers, Young, Kakuma, et al., 1997; Hickie & Scott, 1998). This late-onset depression profile of presumed organic etiology is associated with such symptoms as psychomotor retardation, apathy, extrapyramidal signs, and poor performance on neuropsychological tests of frontal functioning (Simpson, Baldwin, Jackson, & Burns, 1998). This type of depression, moreover, tends to be chronic and treatment-resistant. In a similar manner, another late-onset depression of organic etiology may represent a prodrome of Alzheimer's disease.

Independent of questions regarding the potential organic etiology of depressive symptoms, older patients with depression may exhibit subtly different symptom profiles than do younger patients with depression. Gatz and Fiske (2003) noted that older adults are less likely than are younger adults to report symptoms of dysphoria and guilt, and are more likely to report other symptoms of depression. One common depressive profile among aging adults includes symptoms of anergia, loss of interest, hopelessness, helplessness, and psychomotor retardation. This symptom profile, labeled the *depletion syndrome* (Newmann, Engel, & Jensen, 1991) or *motivation symptom cluster* (Forsell, Jorm, & Winblad, 1994), appears to be more prevalent in older females. In addition, older females with depression are less likely to display direct suicidal attempts and more likely to display indirect suicidal behaviors, such as persistent refusals to eat, drink, or take needed medications (Osgood, Brant, & Lipman, 1991).

Older women report such somatic symptoms as disruptions in sleep, appetite, and sexual interest at particularly high rates (Berry, Storandt, & Coyne, 1984; Bolla-Wilson & Bleecker, 1989; Christensen et al., 1999). This elevated rate of somatic symptom reporting, however, highlights another diagnostic challenge with respect to assessing depression in aging patients—that is, issues relating to increased rates of physical symptoms associated with medical comorbidities. As discussed by Gatz and Fiske (2003), one's health status may affect depressive symptom reporting in a number of ways. To begin, physical problems associated with medical illness or impairment may inflate somatic depression scale scores among patients who are not, in fact, clinically depressed. The fact that increasing health problems are themselves risk factors for depression complicates attempts to tease out this potential bias in reporting among older patients. Physiological effects of medical illness and side effects of pharmacologic treatments for medical ailments may directly affect depressive symptom reports. In addition, medical illness, medical treatments, and associated pain or physical dysfunction may act as discrete or chronic life stressors precipitating depressive episode onset. Research specifically indicates that functional limitations associated with medical illness may be a central factor in explaining this health–depression relationship (Zeiss, Lewinsohn, & Rohde, 1996). The physical limitations and extensive medication regimens of older adults with medical comorbidities, as well as the potential for drug interactions, can add a layer of complexity to the use of antidepressant treatments in this population.

Other specific risk factors for late-life depression in women may include caregiving activities for physically or cognitively disabled spouses or partners (as discussed in the previous section), stressors associated with changes in residence, retirement,

declining financial security, and the increased risk of bereavement among aging women. Bereavement is known to increase
the risk of depressive symptoms, MDD, and anxiety symptoms
and disorders. Moreover, recent research suggests that up to 20%
of bereaved individuals may experience what has been labeled
traumatic grief. As measured with the Inventory of Complicated
Grief (ICG; Prigerson et al., 1995), symptoms of complicated or
traumatic grief may include a preoccupation with thoughts of
the deceased, distressing memories of the deceased, anger, disbe-
lief, an inability to accept the death, difficulties trusting or caring
about others, loneliness, emptiness, bitterness, and avoidance
of—or preoccupation with—reminders of the deceased (see also
Prigerson et al., 1999). Research with the ICG indicates that individuals identified as complicated grievers are more likely than
uncomplicated grievers to report poorer medical health, poorer
mental health, increased pain, increased depressive symptoms,
and poorer social functioning. Older bereaved individuals with
high ICG scores are, moreover, twice as likely to report suicidal
ideation as are those without symptoms of complicated grief
(Prigerson et al., 1997, 1999). Identification and targeted intervention of these older bereaved patients at risk represents a significant public health concern.

Recent reviews (Gerson, Belin, Kaufman, Mintz, & Jarvik, 1999;
Niederehe & Schneider, 1998) support the efficacy of antidepressant medications or psychotherapy or both in the treatment of
older people with depression. As reviewed by Gatz and Fiske
(2003), two studies are of particular note. In the first, Thompson,
Coon, Gallagher-Thompson, Sommer, and Koin (2001) compared
CBT, desipramine, and combined CBT and drug in the acute
treatment of depression among older patients. Posttreatment
outcomes indicated that both CBT and combined treatment were
superior to drug treatment alone, with a trend for combined
treatment to be superior to CBT alone for severe depression. In
the second study, a placebo-controlled study of maintenance
psychotherapy in late-life depression, patients older than 59
years with a clear history of recurrent unipolar depression were
treated to full recovery with open treatment of nortriptyline and
IPT. Recovered subjects were then randomized into one of four
maintenance treatment conditions: monthly maintenance IPT

sessions alone (with placebo), nortriptyline alone (with monthly medication clinic), combined IPT and nortriptyline, or a no-treatment control (placebo and medication clinic). Results indicated that all three active treatments were significantly better than placebo in preventing depression recurrence. Though the preventive capacity of medication alone and maintenance IPT alone did not significantly differ, combined IPT and medication treatment showed a trend toward added benefit over either treatment alone in preserving recovery. This effect was particularly notable in patients 70 years and older (Reynolds et al., 1999).

Chronic Depression

Characterized by prolonged episodes of illness and incomplete remission lasting 2 years or longer, up to one third of depressed patients experience chronic forms of depression (Keller & Hanks, 1994). As reviewed by Kornstein (2002), chronic forms of depression may include chronic major depressive disorder (MDD of at least 2 years duration), dysthymic disorder (chronic mild depression of at least 2 years duration), double depression (MDD superimposed on an episode of dysthymia), and recurrent major depressive disorder with incomplete interepisode recovery.

Patients with chronic depression display a more severe course than do those with more acute or episodic forms of this disorder, including an earlier onset, more suicide attempts, greater psychiatric comorbidities, and more lifetime psychiatric hospitalizations (Keller, Gelenberg, et al., 1998; Klein et al., 1998). Chronic forms of depression are also associated with a poorer treatment response, including a longer time to remission or incomplete symptom response with antidepressant treatments (Harrison & Stewart, 1993; Howland, 1991; Keller, Lavori, Endicott, Coryell, & Klerman, 1983; Koran et al., 2001; Rush & Thase, 1997).

It is not surprising that chronic forms of depression are also associated with particularly severe levels of impairment within social, occupational, and physical domains. Indeed, the impairment associated with depression surpasses that seen in patients with other chronic medical disorders, such as hypertension, arthritis, or diabetes (Hays, Wells, Sherbourne, Rogers, & Spritzer,

1995; Wells, Burnam, Rogers, Hays, & Camp, 1992). It is notable that Kornstein (2002) pointed out that when women become chronically depressed, they fare significantly worse than do their chronically depressed male counterparts. In specific terms, women with chronic forms of depression report greater symptoms, a younger age of illness onset, poorer social adjustment, and a poorer quality of life than do males with chronic depression (Kornstein et al., 2000a). Moreover, results of one study indicated that early-onset depressive disorder adversely affected the lifetime educational attainment of women but not that of men (Berndt et al., 2000).

As reviewed by Kornstein (2002), numerous randomized controlled trials have demonstrated the acute-phase efficacy of several antidepressant medications among chronically depressed patients. Subsequent decreases in depressive symptoms have been associated with improvements in psychosocial functioning among chronically depressed patients, an effect that is particularly clear among those patients who achieve full symptom remission (Miller et al., 1998; Thase et al., 1996). However, patients with chronic forms of depression clearly require a long-term approach to treatment and disease management. Three published studies of chronic depression have shown the effectiveness of antidepressant therapies as long-term maintenance treatments (Gelenberg et al., 2003; Keller, Gelenberg, et al., 1998; Keller, Kocsis, et al., 1998; Kocsis et al., 1996).

As Kornstein (2002) noted, few large-scale trials have examined the efficacy of psychotherapy—either alone or in combination with antidepressants—for the treatment or long-term management of chronically depressed patients. Recent studies support the effectiveness of combined treatments for this population, including the combination of sertraline and IPT (Steiner et al., 1998) and the combination of sertraline and CBT (Ravindran et al., 1999) for dysthymic patients, and the combination of nefazodone and cognitive–behavioral analysis for patients with chronic major depression, double depression, or recurrent major depression with incomplete interepisode recovery (Keller et al., 2000). In the latter study, combination treatment showed a significant improvement in outcome as compared with either psychotherapy or medication treatment alone.

Few studies have evaluated gender differences in antidepressant treatment response among chronically depressed patients. In one 12-week study comparing sertraline, imipramine, and placebo in 410 dysthymic patients, Yonkers et al. (1996) found that more women than men responded to sertraline (64% vs. 42%). In another 12-week study comparing sertraline and imipramine in 635 patients with chronic major or double depression (Kornstein et al., 2000b), women responded more favorably to sertraline than to imipramine (57% vs. 46%) whereas men responded more favorably to imipramine than to sertraline (62% vs. 45%). Illustrating the importance of analyzing treatment outcome data by gender, in both of these studies overall analysis showed no differences in medication response rates.

For females, menopausal status may also influence treatment outcome. For example, Kornstein et al. (2000b) found that whereas premenopausal women responded better to sertraline than to imipramine (57% vs. 43%), there was no difference in response rates to sertraline and imipramine in postmenopausal women (57% vs. 56%). This increased efficacy of the SSRIs among premenopausal women has been clinically noted elsewhere and needs further evaluation. Furthermore, among premenopausal women with chronic depression, existing data suggest that up to 25% may experience a premenstrual exacerbation of mood symptoms (Kornstein et al., 1996), which may also respond to SSRI treatment. Thus, determination of the menopausal status of a woman with chronic depression as well as the potential fluctuation of symptoms across the menstrual cycle may be essential for accurate assessment and treatment.

Recommendations for Research

1. Support research examining the influence of age, puberty, and morphology on gender–mood relationships in adolescents. There are wide methodological variations in the types and reliability of measures used to assess pubertal status, morphological development, and depressive symptoms across existing studies of the adolescent transition. Thus, it is not surprising that attempts to tease out the influence of age, puberty, and morphology on gender–mood relationships during adolescence have resulted in a literature rife with conflicting results. These methodological shortcomings will need to be addressed in future research. In addition, further longitudinal data are needed to track both low- and high-risk males and females across the pubertal transition, to better identify and understand the mechanisms underlying the adolescent onset of the gender gap in depression.

2. *Support research on the adolescent onset of the gender difference in depression.* Future discovery of the biological or psychosocial mechanisms underlying the adolescent onset of the gender difference in depression will go a long way toward guiding the development of targeted interventions to treat and, just as important, to prevent the onset of depressive episodes in females during adolescence and early adulthood. Further research is also needed to determine the effectiveness and feasibility of primary and secondary intervention programs that provide general education for all preadolescents, and more specialized education and intervention for females at high risk. Akin to school-based sex education for adolescents (but, we hope, less controversial), such early mental-health education programs may include dissemination of research-based (yet age-appropriate) information regarding functional versus dysfunctional mood management techniques, as well as general information regarding the symptoms of MDD.

Such educational programs could teach students to identify depression and potential suicidality in peers and provide students with strategies to address these issues and to elicit the aid of parents, teachers, or counselors when appropriate. Well-developed educational programs could help to destigmatize the experience of depression and normalize appropriate treatment-seeking behaviors at an early age, before negative stereotypes regarding psychiatric diagnosis and treatment become entrenched and before ongoing depression can exact the huge toll that it does in this critical period of learning and social development. In light of the close interpersonal relationships often seen among adolescent female peer groups, eliciting female peers to help identify early symptoms of depression and reinforce treatment-seeking behaviors may lead to an increase in the early identification of and effective intervention for this disorder.

3. Focus research efforts on treatment of depression during pregnancy and postpartum. Further research is clearly needed to identify safe and effective treatments for women experiencing depressive episodes during pregnancy and postpartum. To improve informed treatment decision making, further education must be provided to both depressed women and their care providers regarding the pertinent benefits and risks of depression treatment during pregnancy and postpartum. Research is also needed to better determine and characterize the potential risks related to fetal exposure to the physiologic dysregulation of depression during pregnancy. Further research regarding the risks and benefits of pharmacologic agents, as well as the potential role of alternative nonpharmacologic depression treatments, such as light therapy, is needed. Continued development of and research on population-specific psychotherapies that help women adapt to the demands of pregnancy and motherhood are also required. Finally, the field would benefit from research designed to examine risk perception and clinical decision making for pregnant and postpartum patient populations and their primary care providers.

4. Provide more detailed information on the risks of antidepressant use by pregnant and lactating women. There is currently a crucial need for improved FDA pregnancy and lactation risk categories that more accurately reflect the reproductive risks of alternate antidepressant medications. It has been argued that clinicians making treatment decisions based on the current categories alone are likely to overestimate reproductive risks and fail to provide what may represent beneficial and relatively safe depression treatments. This problem and the lack of education among primary care providers regarding empirically based estimates of fetal risk likely contribute to the large proportion of depressed women who go untreated or undertreated during pregnancy and the postpartum period.

5. Encourage prevention and intervention efforts for depressed women with children. Despite the extensive negative impact of depression on both women and their children and the availability of effective treatments, a majority of women with depression and their at-risk children remain untreated. The findings reviewed by Weissman and Jensen (2002) support efforts aimed at the early detection of and intervention for depressed mothers and their at-risk offspring across multiple treatment settings, including pediatric, OB/GYN, and primary care facilities where women and their children are typically seen.

Weissman and Jensen (2002) identified numerous gaps in the research regarding depressed women and their children. To begin, research is needed to determine whether the early detection and treatment of maternal depression will lead to improved psychiatric and functional outcomes among their at-risk offspring. More research on psychotherapeutic and pharmacologic interventions for children and adolescents with depression, as well as research to determine the potential impact of such interventions on long-term mental health and quality of life, is urgently needed. Finally, in light of the significant number of mothers and children with depression who remain untreated or undertreated, there is a need for health services research examining common barriers to care and potential interventions to improve current clinical practice across a variety of practice settings.

One major barrier to care for depressed mothers and their children includes current inadequacies in the dissemination of efficacious depression treatment options. Another major barrier to care lies in the current lack of parity in health coverage currently devoted to mental health, as compared with general health services. Continued efforts to pass and effect parity legislation designed to provide coverage for mental illness on the same basis as for other general medical illness is needed (see Weissman & Jensen, 2002).

6. *Support research on treatment for severe PMS and PMDD.* Despite evidence that supports the efficacy of SSRIs for severe PMS or PMDD, less than 3% of women receive this treatment (Campbell et al., 1997; Hylan et al., 1999; Singh, Berman, Simpson, & Annechild, 1998). In contrast, community studies indicate that women with premenstrual complaints are more likely to try over-the-counter medications, vitamins, or herbal remedies, or to be prescribed nonsteroidal anti-inflammatory drugs and hormonal preparations—treatments for which efficacy data are poor or inconsistent (Campbell et al., 1997; Corney & Stanton, 1991; Hylan et al., 1999; Johnson et al., 1988; Singh et al., 1998).

Yonkers et al. (2003) suggested a number of steps to redress this obvious gap between research findings and the current clinical reality of treating women with PMS or PMDD. First, these authors highlighted the need for effectiveness research to assess existing therapeutic interventions with clinical samples that include women with both syndromal and subsyndromal PMDD symptomatology, as well as patients with co-occurring medical and psychiatric conditions. These studies should be performed within the context of clinical practice settings in which women typically seek care, such as OB/GYN or primary care settings. Finally, research that examines long-term outcomes (e.g., following patients for longer than the typical one to three menstrual cycles) and expands treatment outcomes of interest to include the assessment of functioning and quality of life is needed (see Yonkers et al., 2003).

7. *Expand depression research to include a focus on perimenopause.* Further identification and examination of the subgroup of women with a lifetime history of MDD who may be at heightened risk for depression recurrence or exacerbation during perimenopause (as well as during other periods of intense hormonal fluctuation, such as the postpartum period) is warranted. Further research on the potential role of hormonal fluctuations on mood, as well as novel interventions to treat or prevent mood episodes during these life periods, is also needed.

8. *Develop methods for early identification of and interventions for women in caregiving roles at risk for depression.* Although hindered by the limited proportion of male primary adult caregivers, future prospective research on gender differences in adult caregiver stress and its relationship to increased depression rates is warranted. Early identification of and interventions for at-risk female caregivers may help to prevent or reduce psychiatric morbidity and to facilitate adaptive coping strategies in this population. Further treatment development and intervention research is clearly needed to target this particularly at-risk group.

9. *Improve detection and treatment of depression in aging women.* As noted by Gatz and Fiske (2003), access to mental health care represents a significant issue for many financially strained or physically disabled older women. Improving the detection and effective treatment of depression within primary care settings via

physician education on depression in older people and current treatment guidelines may help to alleviate this problem. Yet, in light of time constraints of primary care physicians and the barriers that may impede older people from seeking or receiving specialized psychiatric care, alternative solutions to meet the mental health needs of older patients with depression should be tested. Such alternatives may include improving the process of referral to specialty care and training nurses or other health care extenders to act within the primary care setting. These care providers may be trained to conduct depression screenings, promote physician adherence to treatment guidelines, provide patient and family psychoeducation about depression, and build networks for referral to specialized care.

10. *Focus detection and intervention efforts to reduce the onset, chronicity, and recurrence of depression in young women.* Accurate and consistent methodological distinctions among the various forms of chronic depression remain a challenge. In clinical settings, such diagnostic distinctions are typically based on retrospective patient reports of the previous 2 years, which may be vague or biased by current mood symptoms. In addition, changes in criteria for the chronic depression subtypes from the *DSM–III–R* to the *DSM–IV* contribute to inconsistencies in the existing literature (Kornstein, 2002).

The severity and impairment associated with chronic depressions, as well as data indicating that women are more adversely affected by chronic depression than are men, warrant early detection and treatment designed to reduce the onset, chronicity, and recurrence of this illness in young women. Chronic forms of depression are especially likely to go unrecognized and untreated. Because of the long-standing nature of these disorders and relative lack of nondepressed baselines for comparison, chronically depressed women (and their friends and family) may be least likely to identify their illness and to seek (or encourage) treatment. As Kornstein (2002) pointed out, increased education for both potential patients and care providers is sorely needed to address this underrecognized and undertreated problem.

In addition, therapeutic strategies designed to bolster the effectiveness of existing treatments for chronically depressed patients are particularly needed in light of the risk associated with residual depressive symptoms that are often observed among chronically depressed patients at posttreatment. Additional strategies designed to obtain complete symptom remission among these patients may include the development of specific psychotherapeutic techniques tailored to meet the needs and challenges of chronically depressed patients, such as recent adaptations of CBT (McCullough, 2000) and IPT (Markowitz, 2003) for chronic depression. Finally, increased development and study of long-term intervention and prevention strategies that combine longer term psychotherapies and antidepressant medications are needed.

Recommendations for Practice and Policy

Beginning at puberty and extending into older age, women are twice as likely as men to experience a lifetime episode of depression. This chapter highlights existing research on various at-risk populations of women and espoused a life span development framework to review a number of literatures regarding depression risk and female reproductive status events, as well as depression risk associated with social or developmental life challenges that many women will face across the life span. However, depression should not be considered a normal part of women's lives. Instead, depression is a chronic or chronically recurrent illness that can rob women of their functioning, economic resources, and emotional quality of life. Research indicates that women's depression risk may be associated with certain reproductive events and with certain life stressors that are more often faced by women (such as sexual abuse or adult caregiving demands).

Failure to treat women with depression has significant ramifications not only for the women themselves but also for their partners, children, families, and communities. Yet, the unfortunate reality is that in a majority of cases this disorder goes undetected, untreated, or seriously undertreated. This reality is all the more lamentable because of the existence of depression treatments that work, and, more specifically, treatments that work within a variety of the targeted populations described above, such as women with PMDD, depressed women who are pregnant or lactating, women with chronic depressions, and older women. Moreover, evidence indicates that if practitioners provide sufficient doses of maintenance treatment (which may include pharmacologic and psychotherapeutic treatments) and appropriate chronic disease management strategies, depression recurrence could be eliminated or significantly reduced, thereby increasing the functioning and quality of life of those women with a lifetime depression history.

A number of general implications regarding treatment, prevention, service delivery, and mental health policy may be gathered from the review in this chapter. First, clinicians need to be alert to the importance of early detection and effective treatment of depression in women and be active in educating various groups of consumers. These groups include the public (women themselves), primary care providers, obstetricians, gynecologists, pediatricians, nurses, and school counselors. In addition, the current review highlights the need for practitioners to provide both adequate and accessible mental health treatments by (a) ensuring that appropriate dosages of effective medications and psychotherapies are provided, (b) paying attention to potential gender differences in treatment adherence and response, (c) understanding the potential influence of the menstrual cycle and reproductive status events on depressive symptoms and treatment response, and (d) working to bring effective treatments to places where women can have access to them easily.

To implement the provision and to enhance the accessibility of depression treatments across these targeted populations, continued efforts to achieve parity in mental health coverage—such as legislative and consumer-based health care policy that strives to place mental health care financing on a similar footing with physical health care financing—are sorely needed (see Weissman & Jensen, 2002). On economic grounds alone, the need for such parity in health care policy is underscored by the recent Global Burden of Disease Study and its projections, as noted in chapter 2 (this volume), that by the year 2020 unipolar major depression will rank second only to ischemic heart disease in terms of global disease burden (Murray & Lopez, 1996).

The topics covered in this review suggest a number of research directions to pursue in the next 5 years. As covered in chapter 1 (this volume), research designed to gain a better understanding of the etiology and mechanisms underlying the gender difference in lifetime depression rates is critical, as such information may have a significant impact on future treatment development and research. In addition, there is a need to examine potential gender effects in depression risk and treatment outcome. Because of the often modest size of depression treatment studies and the underrepresentation of males in many of these data sets, efforts to examine gender differences in combined data sets and in large-scale, multicenter trials may best resolve these questions. To further this goal, grant money to support ancillary studies to existing National Institute of Mental Health multicenter depression treatment trials would enable sophisticated analyses with adequate power to test for such gender differences.

Creative research on depression prevention, based on screening of vulnerable and already ill populations targeted in this review and including stepped interventions for PMDD, pregnancy, postpartum, and chronic depression, is also indicated. Another theme emerging from the current review is that converging data indicate the existence of a subgroup of women who are at particular risk for depressive recurrence or exacerbation during periods of reproductive hormone fluctuation (i.e., during premenstrual, postpartum, and menopausal transitions). Further identification and study of this potential subgroup of at risk women is needed. Finally, further support is needed for treatment trials that move in the direction of effectiveness research—trials that expand entry criteria, expand outcomes of interest, promote the assessment of patient needs and preferences, and tailor treatments for implementation in real-world settings (see Yonkers et al., 2003).

Professional associations as well as federal and state health care agencies could play a major role in both broad-based educational efforts and policy reform measures designed to enhance the identification, prevention, and treatment of depression in women. To begin, these organizations could stimulate collaborative efforts among clinical and health care policy organizations (such as the American Psychological Association, the American

Psychiatric Association, the National Association of Social Workers, and national associations for nurses, physician assistants, and other health care professionals) to increase education and training in empirically based depression treatments and women-focused interventions, and to continue to encourage health care policy reform aimed at increasing access to these treatments for a variety of the targeted populations reviewed. In specific terms, the organizations must correct the assumption that all or most women will have the access or inclination to obtain depression treatments within psychiatric specialty settings by working to move depression treatments to settings where women are likely to go.

Stigma regarding depression and its treatment persists. Therefore, a major role of professional groups and governmental agencies may be an educational one, designed to provide information to women regarding this common disorder, its potential negative ramifications, and effective treatments. Such educational campaigns could be specifically designed to address the prevalence, symptoms, and concerns of targeted groups of women, with marketing strategies that reach these groups in places that they frequent or where they typically receive care. To best tailor these strategies and decrease stigma within these targeted groups, further empirical study will be necessary to better understand the multiple barriers to care faced by these targeted populations, and how best to diminish those barriers to better disseminate appropriate depression treatment and, ultimately, increase women's quality of life.

References

Alexopoulos, G. S., Meyers, B. S., Young, R. C., Campbell, S., Silbersweig, D., & Charlson, M. (1997). 'Vascular depression' hypothesis. *Archives of General Psychiatry, 54,* 915–922.

Alexopoulos, G. S., Meyers, B. S., Young, R. C., Kakuma, T., Silbersweig, D., & Charlson, M. (1997). Clinically defined vascular depression. *American Journal of Psychiatry, 154,* 562–565.

Altshuler, L. L., Cohen, L. S., Moline, M. L., Kahn, D. A., Carpenter, D., & Docherty, J. P. (2001). The Expert Consensus Guideline Series: Treatment of depression in women. *Postgraduate Medicine,* (Spec. No.), 1–107.

American Psychiatric Association. (1994). *Diagnostic and statistical manual of mental disorders* (4th ed.). Washington, DC: Author.

Angold, A., & Rutter, M. (1992). Effects of age and pubertal status on depression in a large clinical sample. *Developmental Psychopathology, 4*, 5–28.

Angold, A., Worthman, C., & Costello, E. (1997, March). *Puberty and depression: A longitudinal epidemiological diagnostic study.* Paper presented at the annual meeting of the American Psychopathological Association, New York, NY.

Appleby, L., Warner, R., Whitton, A., & Faragher, B. (1997). A controlled study of fluoxetine and cognitive–behavioral counseling in the treatment of postnatal depression. *British Medical Journal, 314*, 932–936.

Avis, N. E. (2003). Depression during the menopausal transition. *Psychology of Women Quarterly, 27*, 91–100.

Avis, N. E., Brambilla, D., McKinlay, S. M., & Vass, K. (1994). A longitudinal analysis of the association between menopause and depression: Results from the Massachusetts Women's Health Study. *Annals of Epidemiology, 4*, 214–220.

Bakan, D. (1996). *The duality of human existence: Isolation and communion in Western man.* Boston: Beacon Press.

Baker-Miller, J. (1986). *Toward a new psychology of women.* Boston: Beacon Press.

Bebbington, P. E., Dunn, G., Jenkins, R., Lewis, G., Brugha, T., Farrell, M., & Meltzer, H. (1998). The influence of age and sex on the prevalence of depressive conditions: Report from the National Survey of Psychiatric Morbidity. *Psychological Medicine, 28*, 9–19.

Berndt, E. R., Koran, L. M., Finklestein, S. N., Gelenberg, A. J., Kornstein, S. G., Miller, I. M., et al. (2000). Lost human capital from early-onset chronic depression. *American Journal of Psychiatry, 157*, 940–947.

Berry, J. M., Storandt, M., & Coyne, A. (1984). Age and sex differences in somatic complaints associated with depression. *Journal of Gerontology, 39*, 465–467.

Bolla-Wilson, K., & Bleecker, M. L. (1989). Absence of depression in elderly adults. *Journal of Gerontology, 44*, 53–55.

Bromberger, J. T., Meyer, P. M., Kravitz, H. M., Sommer, B., Cordal, A., Powell, L., et al. (2001). Psychologic distress and natural menopause: A multiethnic community study. *American Journal of Public Health, 91*, 1435–1442.

Brooks-Gunn, J., & Warren, M. P. (1989). Biological and social contributions to negative affect in young adolescent girls. *Child Development, 60*, 40–55.

Brown, G. W., & Harris, T. O. (1978). *The social origins of depression: A study of psychiatric disorder in women.* London: Tavistock.

Burke, K. C., Burke, J. D., Rae, D. S., & Regier, D. A. (1991). Comparing age at onset of major depression and other psychiatric disorders by birth cohorts in five US community populations. *Archives of General Psychiatry, 48*, 789–795.

Burton, L. C., Newson, J. T., Schulz, R., Hirsch, C. H., & German, P. S. (1997). Preventative health behaviors among spousal caregivers. *Preventative Medicine, 26,* 162–169.

Campbell, S. (1976). Double blind psychometric studies on the effects of natural estrogens on postmenopausal women. In S. Campbell (Ed.), *The management of the menopause and postmenopausal years* (pp. 149–158). Lancaster, PA: MTP Press.

Campbell, E. M., Peterkin, D., O'Grady, K., & Sanson-Fisher, R. (1997). Premenstrual symptoms in general practice patients: Prevalence and treatment. *Journal of Reproductive Medicine, 42,* 637–646.

Chambers, C. D., Johnson, K. A., Dick, L. N., Felix, R. J., & Jones, K. L. (1996). Birth outcomes in pregnant women taking fluoxetine. *New England Journal of Medicine, 335,* 1010–1015.

Christensen, H., Jorm, A. F., MacKinnon, A. J., Korten, A. E., Jacomb, P. A., Henderson, A. S., & Rodgers, B. (1999). Age differences in depression and anxiety symptoms: A structural equation modelling analysis of data from a general population sample. *Psychological Medicine, 29,* 325–339.

Cohen, L. S., Soares, C. N., Poitras, J. R., Prouty, J., Alexander, A. B., & Shifren, J. L. (2003). Short-term use of estradiol for depression in perimenopausal and postmenopausal women: A preliminary report. *American Journal of Psychiatry, 160,* 1519–1522.

Collins, A., & Landgren, B. (1995). Reproductive health, use of estrogen and experience of symptoms in perimenopausal women: A population-based study. *Maturitas, 20,* 101–111.

Corney, R. H., & Stanton, R. (1991). A survey of 658 women who report symptoms of premenstrual syndrome. *Journal of Psychosomatic Research, 35,* 471–482.

Cutler, S. E., & Nolen-Hoeksema, S. (1991). Accounting for sex differences in depression through female victimization: Childhood sexual abuse. *Sex Roles, 24,* 425–438.

Cyranowski, J. M., Frank, E., Young, E., & Shear, M. K. (2000). Adolescent onset of the gender difference in lifetime rates of major depression: A theoretical model. *Archives of General Psychiatry, 57,* 21–27.

Dennerstein, L., Smith, A. M. A., Morse, C., Burger, H., Green, A., Hopper, J., & Ryan, M. (1993). Menopausal symptoms in Australian women. *The Medical Journal of Australia, 159,* 232–236.

Epperson, C. N., Terman, M., Terman, J. S., Hanusa, B. H., Oren, D. A., Peindl, K. S., & Wisner, K. L. (2004). Randomized clinical trial of bright light therapy for antepartum depression: Preliminary findings. *Journal of Clinical Psychiatry, 65,* 421–425.

Feingold, A. (1994). Gender differences in personality: A meta-analysis. *Psychological Bulletin, 116,* 429–456.

Ferro, T., Verdeli, H., Pierre, F., & Weissman, M. M. (2000). Screening for depression in mothers bringing offspring for evaluation for treatment of depression. *American Journal of Psychiatry, 157*, 375–379.

Forsell, Y., Jorm, A. F., & Winblad, B. (1994). Association of age, sex, cognitive dysfunction, and disability with major depressive symptoms in an elderly sample. *American Journal of Psychiatry, 151*, 1600–1604.

Frank, E., & Young, E. (2000). Pubertal changes and adolescent challenges: Why rates of depression rise precipitously for girls between ages 10 and 15. In E. Frank (Ed.), *Sex, madness, and society: Gender and psychopathology* (pp. 85–102). Washington, DC: American Psychiatric Press.

Freeman, E. W., Sammel, M. D., Liu, L., Gracia, C. R., Nelson, D. B., & Hollander, L. (2004). Hormones and menopausal status as predictors of depression in women in transition to menopause. *Archives of General Psychiatry, 61*, 62–70.

Gatz, M., & Fiske, A. (2003). Aging women and depression. *Professional Psychology: Research & Practice, 34*, 3–9.

Ge, X., Lorenz, F. O., Conger, R. D., Elder, G. H., & Simons, R. L. (1994). Trajectories of stressful life events and depressive symptoms during adolescence. *Developmental Psychology, 30*, 467–483.

Gelenberg, A. J., Trivedi, M. H., Rush, A. J., Thase, M. E., Howland, R., Klein, D. N., et al. (2003). Randomized, placebo-controlled trial of nefazodone maintenance treatment in preventing recurrence in chronic depression. *Biological Psychiatry, 54*, 806–817.

Gerson, S., Belin, T. R., Kaufman, A., Mintz, J., & Jarvik, L. (1999). Pharmacological and psychological treatments for depressed older patients: A meta-analysis and overview of recent findings. *Harvard Review of Psychiatry, 7*, 1–28.

Halbreich, U., Bergeron, R., Yonkers, K., Freeman, E., Stout, A., & Cohen, L. (2002). Efficacy of intermittent, luteal phase sertraline treatment of premenstrual dysphoric disorder. *Obstetric Gynecology, 100*, 1219–1229.

Halbreich, U., & Smoller, J. W. (1997). Intermittent luteal phase sertraline treatment of dysphoric premenstrual syndrome. *Journal of Clinical Psychiatry, 58*, 1–4.

Hallstrom, T., & Samuelsson, S. (1985). Mental health in the climacteric: The longitudinal study of women in Gothenburg. *Acta Obstetricia et Gynecologica Scandinavica Supplement, 130*, 13–18.

Harrison, W., & Stewart, J. W. (1993). Pharmacotherapy of dysthymia. *Psychiatric Annals, 23*, 638–648.

Hays, R. D., Wells, K. B., Sherbourne, C. D., Rogers, W., & Spritzer, K. (1995). Functioning and well-being outcomes of patients with depression compared with chronic general medical illnesses. *Archives of General Psychiatry, 52*, 11–19.

Hickie, I., & Scott, E. (1998). Late-onset depressive disorders: A preventable variant of cerebrovascular disease? *Psychological Medicine, 28*, 1007–1013.

Holte, A. (1992). A prospective study of healthy Norwegian women. *Maturitas, 14*, 127–141.

Holte, A. (1998). Menopause, mood and hormone replacement therapy: Methodological issues. *Maturitas, 29*, 5–18.

Howland, R. H. (1991). Pharmacotherapy of dysthymia: A review. *Journal of Clinical Psychopharmacology, 11*, 83–91.

Hunter, M. S. (1990). Somatic experience of the menopause: A prospective study. *Psychosomatic Medicine, 52*, 357–367.

Hylan, T., Sundell, K., & Judge, R. (1999). The impact of premenstrual symptomatology on functioning and treatment-seeking behavior: Experience from the United States, United Kingdom, and France. *Journal of Women's Health & Gender-Based Medicine, 8*, 1043–1051.

Istvan, J. (1986). Stress, anxiety, and birth outcomes: A critical review of the evidence. *Psychological Bulletin, 100*, 331–348.

Jermain, D. M., Preece, C. K., Sykes, R. L., & Sulak, P. J. (1999). Luteal phase sertraline for premenstrual dysphoric disorder: Results of a double-blind, placebo-controlled, crossover study. *Archives of Family Medicine, 8*, 328–332.

Joffe, H., Hall, J. E., Soares, C. N., Hennen, J., Reilly, C. J., Carlson, K., & Cohen, L. S. (2002). Vasomotor symptoms are associated with depression in perimenopausal women seeking primary care. *Menopause, 9*, 392–398.

Johnson, S. R., McChesney, C., & Bean, J. A. (1988). Epidemiology of premenstrual symptoms in a nonclinical Sample. 1. Prevalence, natural history and help-seeking behavior. *Journal of Reproductive Medicine, 33*, 340–346.

Kaufert, P. A., Gilbert, P., & Tate, R. (1992). The Manitoba Project: A reexamination of the link between menopause and depression. *Maturitas, 14*, 143–155.

Keller, M. B., Gelenberg, A. J., Hirschfeld, R. M., Rush, A. J., Thase, M. E., Kocsis, J. H., et al. (1998). The treatment of chronic depression, Part 2: A double-blind randomized trial of sertraline and imipramine. *Journal of Clinical Psychiatry, 59*, 598–607.

Keller, M. B., & Hanks, D. L. (1994). The natural history and heterogeneity of depressive disorders. *Journal of Clinical Psychiatry, 56*, 22–29.

Keller, M. B., Kocsis, J. H., Thase, M. E., Gelenberg, A. J., Rush, A. J., Koran, L., et al. (1998, November 18). Maintenance phase efficacy of sertraline for chronic depression: A randomized controlled trial. *Journal of the American Medical Association, 280*, 1665–1672.

Keller, M. B., Lavori, P. W., Endicott, J., Coryell, W., & Klerman, G. L. (1983). "Double depression": Two-year follow-up. *American Journal of Psychiatry, 140*, 689–694.

Keller, M. B., McCullough, J. P., Klein, D. N., Arnow, B., Dunner, D. L., Gelenberg, A. J., et al. (2000). A comparison of nefazodone, the cognitive behavioral-analysis system of psychotherapy, and their combination for the treatment of chronic depression. *New England Journal of Medicine, 342*, 1462–1470.

Kessler, R. C., McGonagle, K. A., Swartz, M., Blazer, D. G., & Nelson, C. B. (1993). Sex and depression in the National Comorbidity Survey I: Lifetime prevalence, chronicity and recurrence. *Journal of Affective Disorders, 29,* 85–96.

Klein, D. N., Norden, K. A., Ferro, T., Leader, J. B., Kasch, K., L., Klein, L. M., et al. (1998). Thirty-month naturalistic follow-up study of early-onset dysthymic disorder: Course, diagnostic stability, and prediction of outcome. *Journal of Abnormal Psychology, 107,* 338–348.

Kocsis, J. H., Friedman, R. A., Markowitz, J. C., Leon, A. C., Miller, N. L., Gniwesch, L., & Parides, M. (1996). Maintenance therapy for chronic depression: A controlled clinical trial of desipramine. *Archives of General Psychiatry, 53,* 769–774, discussion 775–776.

Koran, L. M., Gelenberg, A. J., Kornstein, S. G., Howland, R. H., Friedman, R. A., DeBattista, C., et al. (2001). Sertraline versus imipramine in continuation treatment of chronic depression. *Journal of Affective Disorders, 65,* 27–36.

Kornstein, S. G. (2002). Chronic depression in women. *Journal of Clinical Psychiatry, 63,* 602–609.

Kornstein, S. G., Schatzberg, A. F., Thase, M. E., Yonkers, K. A., McCullough, J. P., Keitner, G. I., et al. (2000a). Gender differences in chronic major and double depression. *Journal of Affective Disorders, 60,* 1–11.

Kornstein, S. G., Schatzberg, A. F., Thase, M. E., Yonkers, K. A., McCullough, J. P., Keitner, G. I., et al. (2000b). Gender differences in treatment response to sertraline versus imipramine in chronic depression. *American Journal of Psychiatry, 157,* 1445–1452.

Kornstein, S. G., Yonkers, K. A., Schatzberg, A. F., Manber, R., & Burke, L. P. (1996, May). *Premenstrual exacerbation of depression.* Paper presented at the American Psychiatric Association 149th Annual Meeting, New York, NY.

Kuh, D. L., Wadsworth, M., & Hardy, R. (1997). Women's health in midlife: The influence of the menopause, social factors and health in earlier life. *British Journal of Obstetrics and Gynaecology, 104,* 923–933.

Kulin, N. A., Pastuszak, A., Sage, S. R., Schick-Boschetto, B., Spivey, G., Feldkamp, M., et al. (1998, February 25). Pregnancy outcomes following maternal use of the new selective serotonin reuptake inhibitors. *Journal of the American Medical Association, 279,* 609–610.

Larson, R., & Richards, M. H. (1989). Introduction: The changing life space of early adolescence. *Journal of Youth and Adolescence, 18,* 501–509.

Larson, R., & Richards, M. H. (1991). Daily companionship in late childhood and early adolescence: Changing developmental contexts. *Child Development, 62,* 284–300.

Lauritzen, C. C. (1973). The management of the pre-menopausal and the postmenopausal patient. In P. A. van Keep & C. Lauritzen (Eds.), *Aging and estrogens.* Basel, Switzerland: Karger.

Lewinsohn, P., Hoberman, H., & Rosenbaum, M. (1988). A prospective study of risk factors for unipolar depression. *Journal of Abnormal Psychology, 97*, 251–264.

Logue, C. M., & Moos, R. H. (1986). Perimenstrual symptoms: Prevalence and risk factors. *Psychosomatic Medicine, 48*, 388–414.

Maccoby, E. (1990). Gender and relationships: A developmental account. *American Psychologist, 45*, 513–520.

Maciejewski, P. K., Prigerson, H. G., & Mazure, C. M. (2001). Sex differences in event-related risk for major depression. *Psychological Medicine, 31*, 593–604.

Mao, K., & Chang, A. (1985). The premenstrual syndrome in Chinese. *Australian and New Zealand Journal of Obstetrics and Gynaecology, 25*, 118–120.

Markowitz, J. C. (2003). Interpersonal psychotherapy for chronic depression. *Journal of Clinical Psychology, 59*, 847–858.

Matthews, K. A., Wing, R. R., Kuller, L. H., Meilahn, E. N., Kelsey, S. F., Costello, E. J., & Caggiula, A. W. (1990). Influences of natural menopause on psychological characteristics and symptoms of middle-aged healthy women. *Journal of Consulting Clinical Psychology, 58*, 345–351.

Mazure, C. M., & Maciejewski, P. K. (2003). A model of risk for major depression: Effects of life stress and cognitive style vary by age. *Depression & Anxiety, 17*, 26–33.

McCullough, J. P. (2000). *Treatment for chronic depression: Cognitive behavioral analysis system of psychotherapy.* New York: Guilford Press.

McKinlay, S. M., Brambilla, D. J., & Posner, J. G. (1992). The normal menopause transition. *Maturitas, 14*, 103–115.

Merikangas, K. R., Foeldenyi, M., & Angst, J. (1993). The Zurich Study. XIX. Patterns of menstrual disturbances in the community: Results of the Zurich Cohort Study. *European Archives of Psychiatry and Clinical Neuroscience, 243*, 23–32.

Miller, I. W., Keitner, G. I., Schatzberg, A. F., Klein, D. N., Thase, M. E., Rush, A. J., et al. (1998). The treatment of chronic depression, Part 3: Psychosocial functioning before and after treatment with sertraline or imipramine. *Journal of Clinical Psychiatry, 59*, 608–619.

Murray, C. J., & Lopez, A. D. (1996, November 1). Evidence-based health policy: Lessons from the Global Burden of Disease Study. *Science, 274*, 740–743.

National Alliance for Caregiving and the American Association of Retired Persons. (1997). *Family caregiving in the US: Findings from a national survey* [Final report]. Bethesda, MD: National Alliance for Caregiving.

Newmann, J. P., Engel, R. J., & Jensen, J. E. (1991). Age differences in depressive symptom experiences. *Journal of Gerontology, 46*, 224–235.

Niederehe, G., & Schneider, L. S. (1998). Treatments for depression and anxiety in the aged. In P. E. Nathan & J. M. Gorman (Eds.), *A guide to treatments that work* (pp. 270–287). New York: Oxford University Press.

Nulman, I., Rovet, J., Stewart, D. E., Wolpin, J., Gardner, H. A., Theis, J. G., et al. (1997). Neurodevelopment of children exposed in utero to antidepressant drugs. *New England Journal of Medicine, 336,* 258–262.

O'Hara, M. W., Neunaber, D. J., & Zekoski, E. M. (1984). Prospective study of postpartum depression: Prevalence, course, and predictive factors. *Journal of Abnormal Psychology, 93,* 158–171.

O'Hara, M., Stuart, S., Gorman, L., & Wenzel, A. (2000). Efficacy of interpersonal psychotherapy for postpartum depression. *Archives of General Psychiatry, 57,* 1039–1045.

Olfson, M., Shea, S., Feder, A., Fuentes, A., Nomura, Y., Gameroff, M., & Weissman, M. M. (2000). Prevalence of anxiety, depression and substance abuse in an urban general medicine practice. *Archives of Family Medicine, 9,* 876–883.

Oren, D. A., Wisner, K. L., Spinelli, M., Eppersen, C. N., Peindl, K. S., Terman, J. S., & Terman, M. (2002). An open trial of morning light therapy for treatment of antepartum depression. *American Journal of Psychiatry, 159,* 666–669.

Osgood, J. J., Brant, B. A., & Lipman, A. (1991). *Suicide among the elderly in long-term care facilities.* New York: Greenwood Press.

Palinkas, L. A., & Barrett-Connor, E. (1992). Estrogen use and depressive symptoms in postmenopausal women. *Obstetrics and Gynecology, 80,* 30–36.

Pastuszak, A., Schick-Boschetto, B., Zuber, C., Feldkamp, M., Pinelli, M., Sihn, S., et al. (1993, May 5). Pregnancy outcome following first-trimester exposure to fluoxetine (prozac). *Journal of the American Medical Association, 269,* 2246–2248.

Paykel, E., Myers, J., Dienelt, M., Klerman, G., Lindenthal, J., & Pepper, M. (1969). Life events and depression: A controlled study. *Archives of General Psychiatry, 21,* 753–760.

Pearce, J., Hawton, K., & Blake, F. (1995). Psychological and sexual symptoms associated with the menopause and the effects of hormone replacement therapy. *British Journal of Psychiatry, 167,* 163–173.

Plouffe, L., Stewart, K., Craft, K. S., Maddox, M. S., & Rausch, J. L. (1993). Diagnostic and treatment results from a southeastern academic center-based premenstrual syndrome clinic: The first year. *American Journal of Obstetrics and Gynecology, 169,* 295–307.

Porter, M., Penney, G. C., Russell, D., Russell, E., & Templeton, A. (1996). A population based survey of women's experience of the menopause. *British Journal of Obstetrics and Gynaecology, 103,* 1025–1028.

Prigerson, H. G., Maciejewski, P. K., Reynolds, C. F., III, Bierhals, A. J., Newsom, J. T., Fasiczka, A., et al. (1995). The Inventory of Complicated Grief: A scale to measure certain maladaptive symptoms of loss. *Psychiatry Research, 59,* 65–79.

Prigerson, H. G., Shear, M. K., Frank, E., Beery, L. C., Silberman, R., Prigerson, J., & Reynolds, C. F., III. (1997). Traumatic grief: A case of loss-induced trauma. *American Journal of Psychiatry, 154,* 1003–1009.

Prigerson, H. G., Shear, M. K., Jacobs, S. C., Reynolds C. F., III, Maciejewski, P. K., Davidson, J. R. T., et al. (1999). Consensus criteria for traumatic grief: A preliminary empirical test. *The British Journal of Psychiatry, 174,* 67–73.

Raffaelli, M., & Duckett, E. (1989). "We were just talking . . .": Conversations in early adolescence. *Journal of Youth and Adolescence, 18,* 567–582.

Ravindran, A. V., Anisman, H., Merali, Z., Charbonneau, Y., Telner, J., Bialik, R. J., et al. (1999). Treatment of primary dysthymia with group cognitive therapy and pharmacotherapy: Clinical symptoms and functional impairments. *The American Journal of Psychiatry, 156,* 1608–1617.

Reynolds, C. F., III, Frank, E., Perel, J. M., Imber, S. D., Cornes, C., Miller, M. D., et al. (1999, January 6). Nortriptyline and interpersonal psychotherapy as maintenance therapies for recurrent major depression: A randomized clinical trial in patients older than 59 years. *Journal of the American Medical Association, 281,* 39–45.

Rivera-Tovar, A. D., & Frank, E. (1990). Late luteal phase dysphoric disorder in young women. *American Journal of Psychiatry, 147,* 1634–1636.

Rush, A. J., & Thase, M. E. (1997). Strategies and tactics in the treatment of chronic depression. *Journal of Clinical Psychiatry, 58*(Suppl. 13), 14–22.

Schmidt, P. J., & Rubinow, D. R. (1991). Menopause-related affective disorders: A justification for further study. *American Journal of Psychiatry, 148,* 844–852.

Schulz, R., O'Brien, A. T., Bookwala, J., & Fleissner, K. (1995). Psychiatric and physical morbidity effects of dementia caregiving: Prevalence, correlates, and causes. *The Gerontologist, 35,* 771–791.

Schulz, R., Visintainer, P., & Williamson, G. M. (1990). Psychiatric and physical morbidity effects of caregiving. *Journal of Gerontology: Psychological Sciences, 45,* 181–191.

Simpson, S., Baldwin, R. C., Jackson, A., & Burns, A. S. (1998). Is subcortical disease associated with a poor response to antidepressants? Neurological, neuropsychological and neuroradiological findings in late life depression. *Psychological Medicine, 28,* 1015–1026.

Singh, B., Berman, B., Simpson, R., & Annechild, A. (1998). Incidence of premenstrual syndrome and remedy usage: A National Probability Sample Study. *Alternative Therapies in Health and Medicine, 4,* 75–79.

Soares, C. N., Poitras, J. R., & Prouty, J. (2003). Effect of reproductive hormones and selective estrogen receptor modulators on mood during menopause. *Drugs & Aging, 20,* 85–100.

Soares, C. N., Poitras, J. R., Prouty, J., Alexander, A. B., Shifren, J. L., & Cohen, L. S. (2003). Efficacy of citalopram as a monotherapy or as an adjunctive treatment to estrogen therapy for perimenopausal and postmenopausal women with depression and vasomotor symptoms. *Journal of Clinical Psychiatry, 64,* 473–479.

Spinelli, M. G. (1997). Interpersonal psychotherapy for depressed antepartum women: A pilot study. *American Journal of Psychiatry, 154,* 1028–1030.

Stattin, H., & Magnusson, D. (1990). *Paths through life: Vol. 2. Pubertal maturation in female development.* Hillsdale, NJ: Erlbaum.

Steiner, M., Browne, G., Roberts, J., Gafni, J., Byrne, C., Bell, B., & Dunn, E. (1998). Sertraline and IPT in dysthymia: One year follow-up. *European Neuropsychopharmacology, 8*(Suppl. 2), S202.

Steiner, M., Korzekwa, M., Lamont, J., & Wilkins, A. (1997). Intermittent fluoxetine dosing in the treatment of women with premenstrual dysphoria. *Psychopharmacology Bulletin, 33,* 771–774.

Stephens, S., & Christianson, J. B. (1986). *Informal care of the elderly.* Lexington, MA: D.C. Heath.

Stewart, D. E., & Boydell, K. M. (1993). Psychologic distress during menopause: Associations across the reproductive life cycle. *International Journal of Psychiatry in Medicine, 23,* 157–162.

Stone, R., Cafferata, G. L., & Sangl, J. (1987). Caregivers of the frail elderly: A national profile. *The Gerontologist, 27,* 616–626.

Sundblad, C., Hedberg, M. A., & Eriksson, E. (1993). Clomipramine administered during the luteal phase reduces the symptoms of premenstrual syndrome: A placebo-controlled trial. *Neuropsychopharmacology, 9,* 133–145.

Swendsen, J. D., & Mazure, C. M. (2000). Life stress as a risk factor for postpartum depression: Current research and methodological issues. *Clinical Psychology: Science and Practice, 7,* 17–31.

Thase, M. E., Fava, M., Halbreich, U., Kocsis, J. H., Koran, L., Davidson, J., et al. (1996). A placebo-controlled, randomized clinical trial comparing sertraline and imipramine for the treatment of dysthymia. *Archives of General Psychiatry, 53,* 777–784.

Thompson, L., Coon, D., Gallagher-Thompson, D., Sommer, B., & Koin, D. (2001). Comparison of desipramine and cognitive/behavioral therapy in the treatment of elderly outpatients with mild-to-moderate depression. *American Journal of Geriatric Psychiatry, 9,* 225–240.

van Keep, P. A., & Kelherhals, J. M. (1974). The impact of sociocultural factors on symptom formation. *Psychotherapy and Psychosomatics, 23,* 251–263.

Warner, V., Weissman, M. M., Fendrich, M., Wickramaratne, P. J., & Moreau, D. (1992). The course of major depression in the offspring of depressed parents. *Archives of General Psychiatry, 49,* 795–801.

Warner, V., Weissman, M. M., Mufson, L., & Wickramaratne, P. J. (1999). Grandparents, parents and grandchildren at high risk for depression: A three-generation study. *Journal of the American Academy of Child & Adolescent Psychiatry, 38,* 289–296.

Weissman, M. M., Bruce, M. L., Leaf, P. J., Florio, L. P., & Holzer, C., III. (1991). Affective disorders. In L. N. Robins & D. A. Regier (Eds.), *Psychiatric disorders in America* (pp. 53–80). New York: Free Press.

Weissman, M. M., Feder, A., Pilowsky, D. J., Olfson, M., Fuentes, M., Blanco, C., et al. (2004). Depressed mothers coming to primary care: Maternal reports of problems with their children. *Journal of Affective Disorders, 78,* 93–100.

Weissman, M. M., & Jensen, P. (2002). What research suggests for depressed women with children. *Journal of Clinical Psychiatry, 63,* 641–647.

Weissman, M. M., Warner, V., Wickramaratne, P., Moreau, D., & Olfson, M. (1997). Offspring of depressed parents 10 years later. *Archives of General Psychiatry, 54,* 932–940.

Wells, K. B., Burnam, M. A., Rogers, W., Hays, R., & Camp, P. (1992). The course of depression in adult outpatients. Results from the Medical Outcomes Study. *Archives of General Psychiatry, 49,* 788–794.

West, C. (1989). The characteristics of 100 women presenting to a gynecological clinic with premenstrual complaints. *Acta Obstetricia et Gynecologica Scandinavica, 68,* 743–747.

Wikander, I., Sundblad, C., Andersch, B., Dagnell, I., Sylberstein, D., Bengtsson, F., & Eriksson, E. (1998). Citalopram in premenstrual dysphoria: Is intermittent treatment during luteal phase more effective than continuous medication throughout the menstrual cycle? *Journal of Clinical Psychopharmacology, 18,* 390–398.

Wisner, K. L., Gelenberg, A. J., Leonard, H., Zarin, D., & Frank, E. (1999, October 6). Pharmacologic treatment of depression during pregnancy. *Journal of the American Medical Association, 282,* 1264–1269.

Wisner, K. L., Parry, B. L., & Piontek, C. M. (2002). Postpartum depression. *The New England Journal of Medicine, 347,* 194–199.

Wisner, K. L., & Perel, J. M. (1988). Psychopharmacologic agents and electroconvulsive therapy during pregnancy and the puerperium. In R. L. Cohen (Ed.), *Psychiatric consultation in childbirth settings* (pp. 165–206). New York: Plenum.

Wisner, K. L., Zarin, D., Holmboe, E., Appelbaum, P., Gelenberg, A. J., Leonard, H., & Frank, E. (2000). Risk-benefit decision-making for treatment of depression during pregnancy. *American Journal of Psychiatry, 157,* 1933–1940.

Woods, N. F., & Mitchell, E. S. (1996). Patterns of depressed mood in midlife women: Observations from the Seattle Midlife Women's Health Study. *Research in Nursing & Health, 19,* 111–123.

Woods, N. F., Most, A., & Dery, G. K. (1982). Prevalence of perimenstrual symptoms. *American Journal of Public Health, 72,* 1257–1264.

Yee, J. L., & Schulz, R. (2000). Gender differences in psychiatric morbidity among family caregivers: A review and analysis. *The Gerontologist, 40,* 147–164.

Yonkers, K. A., Halbreich, U., Rush, A. J., Kornstein, S., Pearlstein, T., & Stone, A. (1996, July). *Sex differences in response to pharmacotherapy among early onset dysthymics.* Paper presented at the annual meeting of the Society for Biological Psychiatry.

Yonkers, K. A., Pearlstein, T., & Rosenheck, R. A. (2003). Premenstrual disorders: Bridging research with clinical reality. *Archives of Women's Mental Health, 6,* 287–292.

Young, S. A., Hurt, P. H., Benedek, D. M., & Howard, R. S. (1998). Treatment of premenstrual dysphoric disorder with sertraline during the luteal phase: A randomized, double-blind, placebo-controlled crossover trial. *Journal of Clinical Psychiatry, 59,* 76–80.

Zeiss, A. M., Lewinsohn, P. M., & Rohde, P. (1996). Functional impairment, physical disease, and depression in older adults. In P. M. Kato & T. Mann (Eds.), *Handbook of diversity issues in health psychology* (pp. 161–184). New York: Plenum.

Zlotnick, C., Johnson, S. L., Miller, I. W., Pearlstein, T., & Howard, M. (2001). Postpartum depression in women receiving public assistance: Pilot study of an interpersonal-therapy-oriented group intervention. *American Journal of Psychiatry, 158,* 638–640.

Chapter

4

Improving Services and Outreach for Women With Depression

Jeanne Miranda

E fficacious treatments for depression are available and, as discussed in previous chapters of this book, include antidepressant medications and brief structured psychotherapies (Schulberg, Katon, Simon, & Rush, 1999; U.S. Department of Health and Human Services, 1999). However, unmet need is common. Less than one quarter of those with depression are

---

Preparation of this chapter was supported, in part, by National Institute of Mental Health Grants MH56864 and MH57909.

As with other chapters in this volume, this integrative review draws heavily on the contributions of all of the participants of the American Psychological Association Summit 2000 on Women and Depression, but especially focuses on the contributions of the following manuscripts: "The Epidemiology of Women and Depression" by Ronald C. Kessler; "The Economics of Depression in Women" by Paul E. Greenberg and Howard G. Birnbaum; "Women With Depression: Changing Barriers to Access" by Sherry Glied; "Women, Depression, and Disability: Exploring the Interconnections" by Judith A. Cook; "Women, Depression, and the Workplace" by Mary Clare Lennon; "Treatment of Ethnically Diverse Women With Depression in Primary Care Settings" by Charlotte Brown; "Cost-Effectiveness of Primary Care Interventions for Depressed Women" by Kathryn Rost; "Assessment and Treatment for Depressed Women in Drug and Alcohol Treatment" by Candace Fleming; and "Improving Services for Women With Anxiety and Depression in Primary Care Settings" by Wayne J. Katon.

likely to get appropriate care (Young, Klap, Sherbourne, & Wells, 2001). To eliminate the excessive burden of depression experienced by women, effective services must be available and engage those who need care.

To be optimally effective, services for women should take into account the prevalence and age of onset of depression, as well as factors associated with risk for depression. In the most recent information on rates of depression in the United States from the National Comorbidity Survey Replication (Kessler et al., 2003), adults in the United States were found to have a lifetime prevalence rate of major depression of 16.2%, with women being 1.7 times more likely than men to experience this disorder. Evidence also suggests that the rates of major depression have increased over the past few decades (Kessler, 2003), indicating the escalating nature of this problem and the urgent need for better care and prevention strategies for women.

Women are more likely than men to have depression, and, as noted in chapter 1 (this volume), this gender difference emerges at early adolescence (Angold, Costello, & Worthman, 1998; Nolen-Hoeksema & Girgus, 1994). This gender disparity is not due to differences in the course of unipolar depression, nor increased recurrence of depression in women compared to men; simply twice as many women as men ever become depressed (Kessler, 2003).

As reviewed by Sinha and Rush in chapter 2 (this volume), depression tends to be a chronic, self-perpetuating disorder (Keller & Hanks, 1994). About 50% of those who experience major depression will recover in a year; however, the risk for recurrence increases with subsequent episodes. Those with multiple prior episodes tend to have worse outcomes than do those experiencing their first episode of depression (Depression Guideline Panel, 1993b).

Socioeconomic Status and Depression

As noted in chapter 1 (this volume), poverty increases the risk for most common mental disorders, including depression

(Dohrenwend & Dohrenwend, 1969, 1974; Holzer et al., 1986; Kessler et al., 1994). Minority women are overrepresented among those who are impoverished (Lamison-White, 1997; see Belle & Doucet, 2003, for a review). Poor mothers with young children have been found to be particularly at risk for depressive symptoms (Belle, Longfellow, & Makosky, 1982; Bogard, Trillo, Schwartz, & Gerstel, 2001; Brown & Harris, 1978; Gyamfi, Brooks-Gunn, & Jackson, 2001). Rates of depression among low-income mothers are nearly twice as high as the general population of women (Bassuk, Buckner, Perloff, & Bassuk, 1998; Miranda & Green, 1999).

Ethnic and Racial Differences in Prevalence

Prevalence rates of depression can vary across racial or ethnic groups in the United States (Brown, Abe-Kim, & Barrio, 2003). The most recent data available on rates of depression across racial or ethnic groups come from the National Comorbidity Survey (NCS; Kessler et al., 1994). In that study, the lifetime rate of depression was 17% for White women, whereas 15% of African American women reportedly experienced an episode of depression at some time in their lives. Although rates of depression for African American and White women are relatively similar, African American women had lower rates of income and were more likely to be impoverished as compared with White women.

Particularly intriguing data on rates of depression in Latina and Asian American women are emerging. For example, rates of depression and substance abuse disorders are low among Mexican Americans born in Mexico (Vega et al., 1998), and immigrant Mexican American women have a lifetime rate of depression of 8%, similar to the rates of nonimmigrant Mexicans (Vega et al., 1998). However, after 13 years in the United States, rates of depression for those women who immigrated to the U.S. rise precipitously. U.S.-born women of Mexican heritage experience lifetime rates of depression similar to those of the White population in the United States, nearly twice the rate of immigrants. These findings are mirrored in other indicators of health. For example, rates of substance abuse disorder and infant mortality rates are similarly low in Mexican-born women but increase with time in the United States (Becerra, Hogue, Atrash, & Perez, 1991). Despite high rates of poverty, Mexican American immigrant women have low rates of physical and mental health problems (Vega et al., 1998). Chinese American immigrant women have a lifetime rate of major depression near 7%, approximately half that of White women (Takeuchi et al., 1998). These results suggest that some aspects of culture may protect against depression. One possible reason for this interesting finding is the difference in cultural social support systems and cultural values of immigrants versus those established in the United States; however, there has been no definitive explanation.

Burden and Cost of Depression

Depression results in enormous personal and societal costs, as noted in the introduction of this book. Depression is a leading cause of disability worldwide (Murray & Lopez, 1996) for a number of reasons. First, as noted, depressive disorders are common, have an early age of onset, and are frequently chronic. Second, depression is highly debilitating. The disability associated with major depression is comparable to that of other medical illnesses such as diabetes or arthritis (Broadhead, Blazer, George, & Tse, 1990; Unützer et al., 2000; Wells et al., 1989), yet the disability tends to occur much earlier in life. A large share of the morbidity is due to reduced productivity at both work and home (Greenberg, Stiglin, Finkelstein, & Berndt, 1993; Sturm, Gresenz, Pacula, & Wells, 1999). For example, major depression is associated with work disability, and treating depression positively affects an individual's capacity to work (Mintz, Mintz, Arruda, & Hwang, 1992). Examining the data from the Epidemiological Catchment Area study, Kouzis and Eaton (2000) found that those with major depression were 2.6 times as likely as their nondepressed counterparts to be receiving disability payments. Furthermore, suicide is associated with depression and is a leading cause of death among adolescents and young adults

(National Health Care Statistics, 1995). Depressive symptoms less severe than major depression are even more common and are also associated with substantial disability (Wells, Sturm, Sherbourne, & Meredith, 1996).

The disability associated with depression cuts across age groups. For example, young people with depression function more poorly in school and social arenas (Asarnow & Ben-Meir, 1988; Kovacs & Goldston, 1991). In later life, depression is also associated with worse quality of life than are a number of chronic medical disorders (Unützer et al., 2000). Cook (2003) summarized the literature, noting that the co-occurrence of depression and disability is overwhelming. Repeated studies have shown higher rates of disability with onset of depression and decreased disability following treatment. Depression also causes disability for subsequent generations. For example, young women who are depressed show marked deficits in parenting (Radke-Yarrow, Cummings, Kuezynski, & Chapman, 1985; Saks et al., 1985; Teti, Gelfand, & Pompa, 1990). Depression affects mother–child interactions, with depressed mothers showing less amicability and emotional expressiveness (Jacob & Johnson, 1997), more negative affect (Goodman, Adamson, Riniti, & Cole, 1994), and more avoidant (Burge & Hammen, 1991) and withdrawn behaviors (Dawson et al., 2003) with their children.

Children of depressed parents function more poorly in academic, social, and mental health areas (Anderson & Hammen, 1993; Gelfand & Teti, 1990) and are nearly three times as likely to become depressed as are children of parents who are not depressed (Birmaher et al., 1996). As a result, depression among mothers is a particularly serious public health problem.

Research is needed to evaluate the cost of depression for women. At the current time, methodological issues remain in terms of measuring the cost of disability for women, particularly for those who are not employed outside of the home (Lennon, 2000). Many studies do not consider the cost associated with a reduction in child and elder care caused by depression in women and may, therefore, underestimate the total burden of depression for women. Furthermore, studies are needed to evaluate the cost of maternal depression as it relates to disability in offspring.

Effective Services for Depression

As noted earlier, effective interventions are available to treat episodes of depression. Both antidepressant medications and brief structured psychotherapies have been shown to improve clinical and functional outcomes (Depression Guidelines Panel, 1993a; Schulberg et al., 1999), and these treatments appear to be effective for diverse populations. For example, a recent study found that these types of interventions were effective for impoverished minority women (Miranda, Azocar, et al., 2003; Miranda, Chung, et al., 2003).

Evidence is also beginning to mount regarding efficacious treatments for dysthymic disorder and minor depression (Akiskal & Cassano, 1997; Harrison & Stewart, 1993; Markowitz, 1994; Miranda & Muñoz, 1994; Szegedi, Wetzel, Angersbach, Philipp, & Benkert, 1997; Williams et al., 2000). Although less robust, some evidence suggests that treatment of depressive symptoms may prevent depressive episodes in adults (Muñoz et al., 1995) and children (Clarke et al., 1995).

Effective strategies are also available for preventing recurrence of depression in those who have suffered multiple episodes of depression. Extended use of antidepressant medications (Frank et al., 1990) and psychotherapy have been shown to prevent recurrence (Blackburn, Eunson, & Bishop, 1986; Evans et al., 1992; Fava, Rafanelli, Grandi, Conti, & Belluardo, 1998; Gortner, Tomas, Gollan, Dobson, & Jacobson, 1998; Teasdale et al., 2001).

Unmet Need for Care

Despite the existence of efficacious interventions, less than half of those who need care actually receive care for depression. In the NCS (Kessler et al., 1994), less than 23% of individuals who had been depressed in the past year had received care from a mental health specialist. Furthermore, only 14% had received treatment from a primary care provider. Though research suggests that antidepressant use has increased dramatically (Olfson, Zarin, Mittman, & McIntyre, 2001), treatment of depression lags far behind its prevalence (Young et al., 2001). Even when any type of care (e.g., clergy, self-help) is included, only 41% of individuals with depression had received help (Kessler et al., 1994).

Of those who do receive care, many fail to receive appropriate care, or care that is consistent with evidence-based guidelines. Young et al. (2001) studied a national community sample of adults who screened positive for depressive or anxiety disorders, and found that about 25% received potentially appropriate care (*Appropriate psychotropic medication* was defined as using the lower end of the therapeutic dosage range for each antidepressant medication as put forth in the Agency for Health Care Policy and Research Guideline for Depression in Primary Care updated for newer medications, and requiring 2 or more months of use during the prior 13 months. *Appropriate counseling* was defined as at least four visits with a mental health specialist or four visits with a primary care practitioner that included counseling for mental health problems). The poor and ethnic minorities are particularly vulnerable to receiving poor-quality care (Young et al., 2001). Zhang, Snowden, and Sue (1998) and Vega, Kolody, Aguilar-Gaxiola, and Catalano (1999) found that Chinese Americans and Mexican Americans are more likely than non-Hispanic Whites to have unmet need for depression care. Young et al. similarly found that African Americans were much less likely than non-Hispanic Whites to receive potentially appropriate care for depression or anxiety.

Women are more likely than men to recognize depressive symptoms, to seek mental health care (Leaf & Bruce, 1987) and to honestly disclose their depressive symptoms (Desai & Jann, 2000). Despite this, most women still do not receive adequate or evidence-based care for depression (Miranda & Green, 1999). However, primary care clinicians are more likely to recognize depression, prescribe antidepressants, and provide guideline-consistent treatment for women than for men (Brown, Shye, & McFarland, 1995; Wang, Berglund, & Kessler, 2000). The research is somewhat less clear regarding ethnic minority women. Earlier research indicated that both recognition (Borowsky et al., 2000) and adequacy of treatment (Brown, Abe-Kim, & Barrio, 2003; Green-Hennessy & Hennessy, 1999; Wang et al., 2000) were substantially lower for ethnic minority women when compared with White women. In a more recent study, Miranda and Cooper

(2004) found that recognition of depression and prescription of appropriate treatment by a primary care doctor did not differ by ethnicity.

Barriers to Care

A range of barriers to depression care has been posited, including financial and time burdens, child-care responsibilities, stigma, lack of information, cultural obstacles, and the disabling aspects of depression (Glied & Kofman, 1995). An important contributor to the financial burden of care is lack of insurance coverage for mental health care. Mental health coverage is a consistently strong predictor of mental health help-seeking, and better insurance coverage is associated with higher levels of use of mental health services (Greenley & Mullen, 1990; Keeler, Manning, & Wells, 1988). In 1999, 18% of adult women between 19 and 64 years of age lacked health insurance (Lambrew, 2001). In fact, the rate of health insurance coverage has declined substantially for women in the past 20 years (Glied, McCormack, & Neufeld, 2003).

Minorities, in particular, have multiple barriers to care. For example, women from cultural backgrounds that emphasize male dominance in family decision making may be unable to attend care without permission of a husband or father (Miranda & Green, 1999). In addition, individuals residing in communities with certain characteristics may be at higher risk for poorer social and health outcomes. Impoverished communities are likely to foster depression as well as provide impediments to depression care such as poor access to quality care and lack of resources for elder and child care. In fact, adverse conditions in communities have been found to increase the risk for health problems above individual risk factors (Coulton, Korbin, Su, & Chow, 1995; Sampson, Morenoff, & Earls, 1999).

Some barriers to care may be specific to women. For example, women who have primary responsibility for child care or elder care may be unable to attend regularly scheduled mental health visits (Miranda & Green, 1999). In addition, young women, those at highest risk for depression, are often not seen in primary care, the setting for much depression care. These women are more likely to be seen in gynecologic and obstetric settings, and limited attention has been paid to addressing care for depression in those settings. Furthermore, as noted earlier, women from cultural backgrounds emphasizing male dominance in family decision making may be unable to attend care without permission of a husband or father (Miranda & Green, 1999), yet the health care system rarely includes family members in treatment planning.

Improving Primary Health Care Services

Almost half of mental health treatment for depressive disorders occurs in primary care systems (Kessler et al., 1994). Young et al. (2001) found that among adults with depression or anxiety, only 20% of those who were seen in a general medical setting were receiving appropriate care, whereas nearly 80% of those seen by a mental health provider were receiving appropriate care.

A number of barriers impede delivery of effective treatment to women with depression in the primary care system. As reviewed by Katon and Ludman (2003), these barriers include competing patient demands; lack of time to provide necessary education and activation of the patient to become a partner in his or her care; infrequent follow-up visits; lack of proactive, objective monitoring of recovery; lack of patient treatment or follow through with referral to the mental health system of care; and lack of access to mental health specialist consultation and feedback because of traditional separation of primary care and mental health systems (Wagner, 1997; Wagner, Austin, & Von Korff, 1996).

Studies have identified a number of factors that are critical to improving the quality of depression care in primary health care settings, including providing support, education, and activation of patients with depression, providing care extenders who support quality care beyond time available from primary care providers, and using monitoring and feedback regarding adherence and outcomes of care to the primary care provider (as reviewed in Katon & Ludman, 2003). Lower cost models using telephone contact to support adherence have resulted in modest gains in levels of appropriate care (Hunkeler et al., 2000; Simon, Von Korff, Rutter, & Wagner, 2000). On the basis of the research findings, Katon and others have recommended a stepped approach to care (moving from lower to higher levels of care on the basis of monitoring outcomes of previous steps, as different people require different levels of care) as the most cost-effective method for treating chronic illness, including depression (Katon, Von Korff, Lin, & Simon, 2001; Von Korff & Tiemens, 2000). Recent studies have evaluated the impact of quality improvement interventions fielded by health care providers using each health care organizations' own staff to provide care (Rost, Nutting, Smith, Werner, & Duan, 2001; Wells et al., 2000). These studies also demonstrate that depression care could be improved largely within existing resources. In one demonstration (Pyne et al., 2000), the improvement in care appeared to be more cost-effective for women than for men. In addition, quality improvement interventions have been shown to benefit ethnic minorities (Miranda et al., 2003) and, in one case, actually eliminate health disparities for minorities (Wells et al., 2004).

Despite the positive results of these trials, interventions to increase quality care for depression have not been widely disseminated. In fact, the available evidence to date suggests that these interventions are not sustained beyond the research study (Lin et al., 1999). In summary, evidence does not suggest that depression care has improved substantially over the past two decades (Ford, 2000).

Financing of Care for Depression

Although many factors have an impact on receipt of quality care for depression, financing of care is critical. National public funding ($35.1 billion in 1996) of mental health care actually exceeds that of private funding ($31.6 billion in 1996; McKusick et al., 1998). However, these systems remain largely underresourced; thus the public system focuses on the most critical cases and is largely geared toward treating those with severe and persistent mental disorders. To curb expenses, private insurance typically provides care for time-limited disorders and shifts responsibility for long-term care to the public sector. As a result, funding has been restricted severely for depressed individuals who are uninsured or covered by Medicaid. Furthermore, many poor young women have only periodic access to Medicaid during pregnancies; they do not have ongoing access to such resources.

In the private sector, limitations on mental health coverage are often apparent. For example, a national survey of employers found that over 90% offered mental health benefits to their employees, but greater than three quarters restricted mental health benefits more severely than they did medical benefits (Buck, Teich, Umland, & Stein, 1997). Over the past decade, policymakers have considered the inequitable coverage of mental disorders. As a result, many states have passed mental health parity legislation. However, this legislation has not resulted in parity (Burnam & Escarce, 1999; Frank & McGuire, 1998). In fact, state parity legislation has had little to no detectable effect on the use of mental health services (Pacula & Sturm, 2000; Sturm & Pacula, 1999). These state laws also do not affect self-insured employers. Furthermore, the emergence of managed care restrains parity by other methods, such as utilization review, formularies, and restricted definitions of medical necessity. Other means of ensuring parity may be necessary to provide quality care for depression to women.

Out-of-pocket expenses that supplement insurance coverage can be prohibitive to those needing depression care. One study (Glied, McCormack, & Neufeld, 2003) examined the out-of-pocket expenses women were required to pay for depression care between 1987 and 1996. During this time, the percentage of out-of-pocket expense for depression care dropped by more than one third, from 41% to 26%. However, care for medical (non–mental health) disorders also fell during this period, reaching 16% by 1996. These data suggest that although out-of-pocket expenditures for depression care for women are becoming lower, this expense is substantially higher than is the expense for medical disorders. As a result, cost is likely to remain a barrier to depression care for many women.

Cost for depression care is also important to employers, as evidenced in recent work of Birnbaum and colleagues (2003). As shown in that study, employers can bear both direct and indirect cost for depression care. Employers can incur direct expenses associated with medical and prescription drug costs stemming from depression care of employees. Further, they can incur the cost of disability claims and illness-related work absences. Birnbaum et al. (2003) found that female and male employees with depression cost more than did their counterparts who did not have depression. A recent study of employer costs found that in 1998, the average employee with depression cost a company approximately $3,000 more per year than did the average beneficiary. These findings clearly suggest that employers would benefit by improving the care their employees receive for depression (Birnbaum et al., 2003).

Recommendations for Research: The Need for Preventive Intervention

1. *Encourage further research on prevention of depression in young women.* The need for preventive interventions to protect women against the excessive morbidity associated with depression is clear. During adolescence, rates of depression accelerate for women, leading to a 2:1 ratio of depression during much of adulthood. Interventions for young girls could potentially prevent onset of the disorder. At the current time, a number of theories have received some support in explaining the gender differences in depression; however, none seems adequate. Though some success in preventing onset of depression has been achieved with cognitive–behavioral interventions for those at high risk for depression (Clarke et al., 1995; Muñoz et al., 1995), further understanding of the factors that lead to high rates of depression for adolescent girls and women could potentially advise preventive interventions.

Data suggest that rates of depression are increasing with each recent decade. However, data from Mexican-born populations, as well as Chinese Americans, suggest that aspects of culture, such as social support systems and values, can protect against depression. Further knowledge of factors associated with low rates of depression among recent immigrants could help to inform effective preventive interventions. Large-scale preventive interventions are clearly needed to lower the excessive morbidity from the rapidly increasing rates of depression in this country.

Despite higher rates of adverse life circumstances, African Americans do not have higher rates of depressive disorders. Research on protective factors, resiliency, and culturally based coping strategies might inform future efforts on developing effective intervention strategies.

As described earlier, effective interventions for depression are available. However, three areas remain problematic. First, efficacy trials have been limited to largely adult White, educated populations who seek psychiatric care. Second, to date, these evidence-based interventions have not been widely available to those with depression. Finally, even fewer individuals adhere to maintenance regimens intended to prevent recurrence of depression.

Although interventions for depression are well established for adults, much less is available for youth. In light of the early onset of depression among adolescent girls, developing interventions for this young population is important such that this population is better able to make critical decisions regarding career and family during critical junctures in their lives. One important focus for interventions for this group should be school settings.

2. *Conduct further research on adapting interventions for ethnic minority populations.* Although evidence is strong regarding the efficacy of both psychotropic and psychotherapeutic interventions for depression, the populations on which these interventions have been based are limited. In a special analysis conducted for the supplement to *Mental Health: A Report of the Surgeon General* entitled *Mental Health: Culture, Race, and Ethnicity* (United States Public Health Service, 2001), the randomized trials of care for depression used by the American Psychiatric Association to develop guidelines for treatment of depression were examined. In that analysis, nearly 4,000 individuals were involved in these clinical trials. Of those, only 29 were identified as specific ethnic minorities. Data on efficacy of these interventions for ethnic minority individuals are clearly lacking. Furthermore, little data are available regarding tailoring depression interventions for ethnic minority populations.

3. *Expand research on effectiveness of care to examine more about outcomes of children of mothers with depression.* The impact on offspring of treating depression in their mothers is not currently

known. In light of the strong link between depression and poor functional and emotional outcome in offspring, learning to decrease these deficits in children through individual or family interventions should be a current priority.

4. *Conduct further research to determine effective means of disseminating depression care information to practitioners and to the public so that young girls and women have access to evidence-based care.* Although interventions are available, little information has been available regarding effective dissemination of these interventions. In specific terms, despite the fact that guidelines are available for treatment of depression, many individuals treated for depression do not receive evidence-based care. New data from the Partners in Care Study (Wells et al., 2000) indicate that care for depression can be established in current health care settings. However, as of yet, the mental health field has not established effective technologies for widely disseminating these interventions to physicians, psychologists, and other health practitioners working in diverse health care settings.

5. *Conduct new research on reducing the stigma associated with seeking care for depression.* Along with improving the availability of care, improving receptivity to care is also important. Community interventions must continue to demonstrate effective ways to educate the public regarding depression and to lower the stigma associated with seeking mental health care. In particular, efforts need to be made to reach communities who are unlikely to receive care, such as ethnic minorities and low-income communities.

6. *Strengthen the important area of community research to further an understanding of those factors within communities that affect depression rates and treatment-seeking.* A particular challenge for community research is gaining an understanding of the impact community factors can have on depression. In light of recent findings that communities can influence rates of mental health beyond individual risk factors (Coulton et al., 1995; Sampson et al., 1999), community-based interventions are potentially important for strengthening communities at risk and decreasing rates of depression.

7. *Develop evidence-based interventions for women with comorbid substance abuse and depression.* Interventions that would meet the

special needs of women with both substance use and mood disorders are needed. These interventions should take into account the needs of women who are currently parenting children. For example, residential treatments may need to provide housing for children as well as the women obtaining care.

Recommendations for Policy

Policy is needed to ensure access to care for women, many of whom have children negatively influenced by ongoing maternal depression. The research findings to date have very clear implications for policy. Poor women who are either uninsured or on Medicaid are unlikely to obtain care for depression within the public sector because limited resources often direct the focus of those services to those with persistent and chronic mental illness. As indicated previously in this volume, depression is a chronic disorder but because of its often episodic course, is frequently not seen as such. Furthermore, many of these women may need assistance with child care, elder care, or transportation. Few resources are currently available to assist low-income women in obtaining care for depression.

Public policy may be necessary to ensure adequate access to depression care within the private sector. Again, mental health parity is critical for increasing access to mental health services because those who benefit most from care (individuals and families) are not those who bear the largest direct percentage of the cost for care (employers and health care organizations). Because of this imbalance, public policy that ensures appropriate access to depression care for all women may be needed.

References

Akiskal, H. S., & Cassano, G. B. (Eds). (1997). *Dysthymia and the spectrum of chronic depression.* New York: Guilford Press.

Anderson, C. A., & Hammen, C. L. (1993). Psychosocial outcomes of children of unipolar depressed, bipolar medically ill, and normal women: A longitudinal study. *Journal of Consulting and Clinical Psychology, 61,* 448–454.

Angold, A., Costello, E. J., & Worthman, C. M. (1998). Puberty and depression: The roles of age, pubertal status, and pubertal timing. *Psychological Medicine, 28,* 51–61.

Asarnow, J., & Ben-Meir, S. (1988). Children with schizophrenia spectrum and depressive disorders: A comparative study of premorbid adjustment, onset pattern, and severity of impairment. *Journal of Child Psychology and Psychiatry, 29,* 477–488.

Bassuk, E., Buckner, J., Perloff, J., & Bassuk, S. (1998). Prevalence of mental health and substance use disorders among homeless and low-income housed mothers. *American Journal of Psychiatry, 155,* 1561–1564.

Becerra, J. E., Hogue, C. J., Atrash, H. K., & Perez, N. (1991, January 9). Infant mortality among Hispanics: A portrait of heterogeneity. *Journal of the American Medical Association, 265,* 217–221.

Belle, D., & Doucet, J. (2003). Poverty, inequality, and discrimination as sources of depression among U.S. women. *Psychology of Women Quarterly, 27,* 101–113.

Belle, D., Longfellow, C., & Makosky, V. P. (1982). Stress, depression and the mother–child relationship: Report of a field study. *International Journal of Sociology of the Family, 12,* 251–263.

Birmaher, B., Ryan, N., Williamson, D., Brent, D., Kaufman, J., Dahl, R., et al. (1996). Childhood and adolescent depression: A review of the past 10 years, Part I. *Journal of the American Academy of Child & Adolescent Psychiatry, 35,* 1427–1439.

Birnbaum, H. G., Leong, S. A., & Greenberg, P. E. (2003). The economics of women and depression: An employer's perspective. *Journal of Affective Disorders, 74,* 15–22.

Blackburn, I. M., Eunson, K. M., & Bishop, S. (1986). A two-year naturalistic follow-up of depressed patients treated with cognitive behavioral therapy, pharmacotherapy, and a combination of both. *Journal of Affective Disorders, 10,* 67–75.

Bogard, C. J., Trillo, A., Schwartz, M., & Gerstel, N. (2001). Future employment among homeless single mothers: The effects of full-time work experience and depressive symptomatology. *Women and Health, 32,* 137–157.

Borowsky, S. J., Rubenstein, L. V., Meredith, L. S., Camp, P., Jackson-Triche, M., & Wells, K. B. (2000). Who is at risk of nondetection of mental health problems in primary care? *Journal of General Internal Medicine, 15,* 381–388.

Broadhead, W., Blazer, D., George, L., & Tse, C. (1990, November 21). Depression, disability days, and days lost from work in a prospective epidemiologic survey. *Journal of the American Medical Association, 264,* 2524–2528.

Brown, C., Abe-Kim, J. S., & Barrio, C. (2003). Depression in ethnically diverse women: Implications for treatment in primary care settings. *Psychology of Women Quarterly, 34,* 10–19.

Brown, G. W., & Harris, T. O. (1978). *The social origins of depression: A study of psychiatric disorder in women.* London: Tavistock.

Brown, J. B., Shye, D., & McFarland, B. (1995). The paradox of guideline implementation: How HCPR's depression guidelines were adapted at Kaiser Permanente Northwest Region. *Journal of Quality Improvement, 21,* 5–21.

Buck, J. A., Teich, J. L., Umland, B., & Stein, M. (1997). Behavioral health benefits in employer-sponsored health plans. *Health Affairs, 18,* 147–157.

Burge, D., & Hammen, C. (1991). Maternal communication: Predictors of outcome at follow-up in a sample of children at high and low risk for depression. *Journal of Abnormal Psychology, 100,* 174–180.

Burnam, M. A., & Escarce, J. J. (1999). Equity in managed care for mental disorders. *Health Affairs, 18,* 22–31.

Clarke, G. N., Hawkins, W., Murphy, M., Sheeber, L. B., Lewinsohn, P. M., & Sheeley, J. R. (1995). Targeted prevention of unipolar depressive disorder in an at-risk sample of high school adolescents: A randomized trial of a group cognitive intervention. *Journal of the American Academy of Child & Adolescent Psychiatry, 34,* 312–321.

Cook, J. (2003). Depression, disability, and rehabilitation services for women. *Psychology of Women Quarterly, 27,* 121–129.

Coulton, C. J., Korbin, J. E., Su, M., & Chow, J. (1995). Community level factors and child maltreatment rates. *Child Development, 66,* 1262–1276.

Dawson, G., Ashman, S. B., Panagiotides, H., Hessl, D., Self, J., Yamada, E., & Embry, L. (2003). Preschool outcomes of children of depressed mothers: Role of maternal behavior, contextual risk, and children's brain activity. *Child Development, 74,* 1158–1175.

Depression Guideline Panel. (1993a). *Depression in primary care: Detection and diagnosis.* Rockville, MD: Agency for Health Care Policy Research.

Depression Guideline Panel. (1993b). *Depression in primary care: Treatment of major depression.* Rockville, MD: Agency for Health Care Policy Research.

Desai, H. D., & Jann, M. W. (2000). Major depression in women: A review of the literature. *Journal of the American Pharmacists Association, 40,* 525–537.

Dohrenwend, B. P., & Dohrenwend, B. S. (1969). *Social status and psychological disorders: A causal inquiry.* New York: Wiley.

Dohrenwend, B. S., & Dohrenwend, B. P. (1974). *Stressful life events: Their nature and effects.* New York: Wiley.

Evans, M. D., Hollon, S. D., De Rubeis, R. J., Piasecki, J. M., Grove, W. M., Garvey, M. J., & Tuason, V. B. (1992). Differential relapse following cognitive therapy and pharmacotherapy for depression. *Archives of General Psychiatry, 49,* 802–808.

Fava, G. A., Rafanelli, C., Grandi, S., Conti, S., & Belluardo, P. (1998). Prevention of recurrent depression with cognitive behavioral therapy: Preliminary findings. *Archives of General Psychiatry, 55,* 816–820.

Fleming, C. M. (2000, October). *Assessment and treatment for depressed women in drug and alcohol treatment.* Paper presented at the American Psychological Association Summit 2000 on Women and Depression, Queenstown, MD.

Ford, D. E. (2000). Managing patients with depression: Is primary care up to the challenge? *Journal of General Internal Medicine, 15,* 344–345.

Frank, E., Kupfer, D. J., Perel, J. M., Corness, C., Jarrett, D. B., Mallinger, A. G., et al. (1990). Three-year outcomes for maintenance therapies in recurrent depression. *Archives of General Psychiatry, 47,* 1093–1099.

Frank, R. G., & McGuire, T. B. (1998). Parity for mental health and substance abuse care under managed care. *Journal of Mental Health Policy and Economics, 1,* 143–159.

Gelfand, D. M., & Teti, D. M. (1990). The effects of maternal depression on children. *Clinical Psychology Review, 10,* 329–353.

Glied, S., & Kofman, S. (1995). *Women and mental health: Issues for health reform.* New York: Commonwealth Fund Commission on Women's Health.

Glied, S., McCormack, S., & Neufeld, A. (2003). Women with depression: Financial barriers to access. *Professional Psychology: Research and Practice, 34,* 20–25.

Goodman, S. H., Adamson, L. B., Riniti, J., & Cole, S. (1994). Mother's expressed attitudes: Associations with maternal depression and children's self-esteem and psychopathology. *Journal of the American Academy of Child & Adolescent Psychiatry, 33,* 1265–1274.

Gortner, G., Tomas, E., Gollan, J. K., Dobson, K. S., & Jacobson, N. S. (1998). Cognitive–behavioral treatment for depression: Relapse prevention. *Journal of Consulting and Clinical Psychology, 66,* 377–384.

Green-Hennessy, S., & Hennessy, K. D. (1999). Demographic differences in medication use among individuals with self-reported major depression. *Psychiatric Services, 50,* 257–259.

Greenberg, P. E., Stiglin, L. E., Finkelstein, S. N., & Berndt, E. R. (1993). The economic burden of depression in 1990. *Journal of Clinical Psychology, 54,* 405–418.

Greenley, J. R., & Mullen, J. (1990). Help-seeking and the use of mental health services. In J. R. Greenley (Ed.), *Research in community and mental health:* (pp. 325–351). Greenwich, CT: JAI Press.

Gyamfi, P., Brooks-Gunn, J., & Jackson, A. P. (2001). Associations between employment and financial and parental stress in low-income single Black mothers. *Women and Health 23,* 119–135.

Harrison, W. M., & Stewart, J. W. (1993). Pharmacotherapy of dysthymia. *Psychiatry Annual, 23,* 638–648.

Holzer, C. E., III, Shea, B. M., Swanson, J. W., Leaf, P. J., Myers, J. K., George, L., et al. (1986). The increased risk for specific psychiatric disorders among persons of low socioeconomic status. *American Journal of Social Psychiatry, 6,* 259–271.

Hunkeler, E. M., Meresman, J., Hargreaves, W. A., Fireman, B., Berman, W. H., Kirsch, A., et al. (2000). Efficacy of nurse telehealth care and peer support in augmenting treatment of depression in primary care. *Archives of Family Medicine, 9,* 700–708.

Jacob, T., & Johnson, S. L. (1997). Parent–child interaction among depressed fathers and mothers: Impact on child functioning. *Journal of Family Psychology, 11,* 391–409.

Katon, W. J., & Ludman, E. J. (2003). Improving services for women with depression in primary care settings. *Psychology of Women Quarterly, 27,* 114–120.

Katon, W., Von Korff, M., Lin, E., & Simon, G. (2001). Rethinking practitioners' roles in chronic illness: The specialist, primary care physician, and the practice nurse. *General Hospital Psychiatry, 23,* 138–144.

Keeler, E. B., Manning, W. G., & Wells, K. B. (1988). The demand for episodes of mental health services. *Journal of Health Economics, 7,* 369–392.

Keller, M. B., & Hanks, D. L. (1994). The natural history and heterogeneity of depressive disorders: Implications for rational antidepressant therapy. *Journal of Clinical Psychiatry, 55*(Suppl. A), 25–31, discussion 32–33, 98–100.

Kessler, R. C. (2003). The epidemiology of women and depression. *Journal of Affective Disorders, 74,* 5–13.

Kessler, R. C., Berglund, P., Demler, O., Jin, R., Koretz, D., Merikangas, K. R., et al. (2003, June 18). The epidemiology of major depressive disorder: Results from the National Comorbidity Survey Replication (NCS–R). *Journal of the American Medical Association, 289,* 3095–3105.

Kessler, R. C., McGonagle, K. A., Swartz, M., Blazer, D. G., & Nelson, C. B. (1993). Sex and depression in the National Comorbidity Survey I: Lifetime prevalence, chronicity and recurrence. *Journal of Affective Disorders, 29,* 85–96.

Kessler, R. C., McGonagle, K. A., Zhao, S., Nelson, C. B., Hughes, M., Eshleman, S., et al. (1994). Lifetime and 12-month prevalence of *DSM–III–R* psychiatric disorders in the United States: Results from the National Comorbidity Survey. *Archives of General Psychiatry, 51,* 8–19.

Kouzis, A. C., & Eaton, W. W. (2000). Psychopathology and the initiation of disability payments. *Psychiatric Services, 51,* 908–913.

Kovacs, M., & Goldston, D. (1991). Cognitive and social cognitive development of depressed children and adolescents. Special section: Longitudinal research. *Journal of the American Academy of Child & Adolescent Psychiatry, 30,* 388–392.

Lambrew, J. M. (2001). *Diagnosing disparities in health insurance for women: A prescription for change.* New York: The Commonwealth Fund.

Lamison-White, L. (1997). *U.S. Bureau of the Census, Current Populations, Series P60-198.* Washington, DC: U.S. Government Printing Office.

Leaf, P. J., & Bruce, M. L. (1987). Gender differences in the use of mental health-related services: A re-examination. *Journal of Health and Social Behavior, 128,* 171–183.

Lennon, M. C. (2000, October). *Women, depression, and the workplace.* Paper presented at the American Psychological Association Summit 2000 on Women and Depression, Queenstown, MD.

Lin, E. H., Simon, G. E., Katon, W. J., Russo, J. E., Von Korff, M., Bush, T. M., et al. (1999). Can enhanced acute-phase treatment of depression improve long-term outcomes? A report of randomized trials in primary care. *American Journal of Psychiatry, 156,* 643–645.

Markowitz, J. C. (1994). Psychotherapy of dysthymia. *American Journal of Psychiatry, 151,* 1114–1121.

McKusick, D., Mark, T. L., King, E., Harwood, R., Buck, J. A., Dilonardo, J., & Genuardi, J. S. (1998). Spending for mental health and substance abuse treatment, 1996. *Health Affairs, 17,* 147–157.

Mintz, J., Mintz, L. I., Arruda, M. J., & Hwang, S. S. (1992). Treatments of depression and the functional capacity to work. *Archives of General Psychiatry, 49,* 761–768.

Miranda, J., Azocar, F., Organista, K. C., Dwyer, E., & Areane, P. (2003). Treatment of depression among impoverished primary care patients from ethnic minority groups. *Psychiatric Services, 54,* 219–225.

Miranda, J., Chung, J. Y., Green, B. L., Krupnick, J., Siddique, J., Revicki, D. A., & Belin, T. (2003, July 2). Treating depression in predominantly low-income young minority women: A randomized controlled trial. *Journal of the American Medical Association, 290,* 57–65.

Miranda, J., & Cooper, L. A. (2004). Disparities in care for depression among primary care patients. *Journal of General Internal Medicine, 19,* 120–126.

Miranda, J., & Green, B. L. (1999). The need for mental health services focusing on poor young women. *Journal of Mental Health Policy Economy, 2,* 73–89.

Miranda, J., & Muñoz, R. (1994). Intervention for minor depression in primary care patients. *Psychosomatic Medicine, 56,* 136–142.

Muñoz, R. F., Ying, Y., Bernal, G., Perez-Stable, E. J., Miranda, J., & Hargreaves, W. (1995). Prevention of depression with primary care patients: A randomized controlled trial. *American Journal of Community Psychology, 23,* 199–222.

Murray, C., & Lopez, A. D. (Eds.). (1996). *The global burden of disease: A comprehensive assessment of mortality and disability from disease, injuries, and risk factors in 1990 and projected to 2020.* Boston: University Press.

National Health Care Statistics. (1995). *Monthly Vital Statistics Report, 43,* 366–369.

Nolen-Hoeksema, S., & Girgus, J. S. (1994). The emergence of gender differences in depression in adolescence. *Psychological Bulletin, 115,* 424–443.

Olfson, M., Zarin, D. A., Mittman, B. S., & McIntyre, J. S. (2001). Is gender a factor in psychiatrists' evaluation and treatment of patients with major depression? *Journal of Affective Disorders, 63,* 149–157.

Pacula, R. L., & Sturm, R. (2000). Mental health parity legislation: Much ado about nothing? *Health Services Research, 35*(1, Pt. 2), 263–275.

Pyne, J. M., Smith, J., Fortney, J., Zhang, M., Williams, D. K., & Rost, K. (2000). Cost-effectiveness of primary care interventions for depressed females. *Journal of Affective Disorders, 74,* 23–32.

Radke-Yarrow, M., Cummings, E. M., Kuezynski, L., & Chapman, M. (1985). Patterns of attachment in two- and three- year-olds in normal families and families with parental depression. *Child Development, 56,* 884–893.

Rost, K., Nutting, P., Smith, J., Werner, J., & Duan, N. (2001). Improving depression outcomes in community primary care practice: A randomized trial of the QUEST intervention: Quality Enhancement by Strategic Teaming. *Journal of General Internal Medicine, 16,* 143–149.

Saks, B. R., Frank, J. B., Lowe, T. L., Berman, W., Naftolin, F., Phil, D., & Cohen, D. J. (1985). Depressed mood during pregnancy and the puerperium: Clinical recognition and implications for clinical practice. *American Journal of Psychiatry, 142,* 728–731.

Sampson, R. J., Morenoff, J. D., & Earls, F. (1999). Beyond social capital: Spatial dynamics of collective efficacy for children. *American Sociological Review, 64,* 633–660.

Schulberg, H. C., Katon, W., Simon, G. E., & Rush, A. J. (1999). Treating major depression in primary care practice. *Archives of General Psychiatry, 55,* 1121–1127.

Simon, G., Von Korff, M., Rutter, C., & Wagner, E. (2000). Randomized trial of monitoring, feedback, and management of care by telephone to improve treatment of depression in primary care. *British Medical Journal, 320,* 550–554.

Sturm, R., Gresenz, C. R., Pacula, R. I., & Wells, K. B. (1999). Labor force participation by persons with mental illness. *Psychiatric Services, 11,* 1407.

Sturm, R., & Pacula, R. L. (1999). State mental health parity laws: Cause or consequence of differences in use? *Health Affairs, 18,* 182–192.

Szegedi, A., Wetzel, H., Angersbach, D., Philipp, M., & Benkert, O. (1997). Response to treatment in minor and major depression: Results of a double-blind comparative study with paroxetine and maprotiline. *Journal of Affective Disorders, 45,* 167–178.

Takeuchi, D. T., Chung, R. C. Y., Lin, K. M., Shen, H., Kurasaki, K., Chun, C. A., & Sue, S. (1998). Lifetime and twelve-month prevalence rates of major depressive episodes and dysthymia among Chinese Americans in Los Angeles. *American Journal of Psychiatry, 155,* 1407–1414.

Teasdale, J. D., Scott, J., Moore, R. G., Hayhurst, H., Pope, M., & Paykel, E. S. (2001). How does cognitive therapy prevent relapse in residual depression? Evidence from a controlled trial. *Journal of Consulting and Clinical Psychology, 69,* 347–357.

Teti, D. M., Gelfand, D. M., & Pompa, J. (1990). Depressed mothers' behavioral competence with their infants: Demographic and psychosocial correlates. *Development and Psychopathology, 2,* 259–270.

United States Public Health Service. (2001). *Mental health: Culture, race, and ethnicity: A supplement to mental health: Report of the Surgeon General.* Washington, DC: Department of Health and Human Services.

Unützer, J., Patrick, D., Diehr, P., Simon, G., Grembowski, D., & Katon, W. (2000). Quality adjusted life years in older adults with depressive symptoms and chronic medical disorders. *International Psychogeriatrics, 12,* 15–33.

U.S. Department of Health and Human Services. (1999). *Mental health: A report of the Surgeon General.* Rockville, MD: U.S. Department of Health and Human Services, Substance Abuse and Mental Health Services Administration, Center for Mental Health Services, National Institutes of Health, National Instutute of Mental Health.

Vega, W. A., Kolody, B., Aguilar-Goxiola, S., Alderete, E., Catalano, R., & Caraveo-Anduaga, J. (1998). Lifetime prevalence of *DSM–III–R* psychiatric disorders among urban and rural Mexican Americans in California. *Archives of General Psychiatry, 55,* 771–778.

Vega, W. A., Kolody, B., Aguilar-Gaxiola, S., & Catalano, R. (1999). Gaps in service utilization by Mexican Americans with mental health problems. *American Journal of Psychiatry, 156,* 928–934.

Von Korff, M., & Tiemens, B. (2000). Individualized stepped care of chronic illness. *Western Journal of Medicine, 172,* 133–137.

Wagner, E. (1997). Managed care and chronic illness: Health services research needs. *Health Services Research, 32,* 702–914.

Wagner, E., Austin, B., & Von Korff, M. (1996). Organizing care for patients with chronic illness. *Milbank Quarterly, 74,* 511–543.

Wang, P. S., Berglund, P., & Kessler, R. C. (2000). Recent care of common mental disorders in the United States: Prevalence and conformance with evidence-based recommendations. *Journal of General Internal Medicine, 15,* 284–292.

Wells, K. B., Sherbourne, C., Schoenbaum, M., Duan, N., Meredith, L., Unützer, J., et al. (2000, January 12). Impact of disseminating quality improvement programs for depression in managed primary care: A randomized controlled trial. *Journal of the American Medical Association, 283,* 212–220.

Wells, K. B., Sherbourne, C., Schoenbaum, M., Ettner, S., Duan, N., Miranda, J., et al. (2004). Five-year impact of quality improvement for depression: Results of a group-level randomized controlled trial. *Archives of General Psychiatry, 61,* 378–386.

Wells, K. B., Stewart, A., Hays, R. D., Burnam, A., Rogers, W., Daniels, M., et al. (1989, August 18). The functioning and well-being of depressed patients: Results from the Medical Outcomes Study. *Journal of the American Medical Association, 262,* 914–919.

Wells, K. B., Sturm, R., Sherbourne, D. C., & Meredith, L. S. (1996). *Caring for depression.* Cambridge, MA: Harvard University Press.

Williams, J. W., Jr., Barrett, J., Oxman, T., Frank, E., Katon, W., Sullivan, M., et al. (2000, September 27). Treatment of dysthymia and minor depression in primary care: A randomized controlled trial in older adults. *Journal of the American Medical Association, 284,* 1519–1526.

Young, A. S., Klap, R., Sherbourne, C. D., & Wells, K. B. (2001). The quality of care for depressive and anxiety disorders in the United States. *Archives of General Psychiatry, 58,* 55–61.

Zhang, A. Y., Snowden, L. R., & Sue, S. (1998). Differences between Asian- and White-Americans' help-seeking and utilization patterns in the Los Angeles area. *Journal of Community Psychology, 26,* 317–326.

Author Index

Numbers in italics refer to listings in the references.

Subject Index

About the Editors

Carolyn M. Mazure, PhD, is a professor of psychiatry and associate dean for faculty affairs at Yale University School of Medicine. Dr. Mazure's research has focused on the development of models for understanding onset and treatment response in depression and, more recently, in addictive disorders. She created and directs Yale's interdisciplinary research program on health and gender, *Women's Health Research at Yale*.

Dr. Mazure came to Yale for her fellowship training after completing graduate school and 3 years at the National Institutes of Health (NIH), where she worked in studies on the genetics of psychiatric disorders. Immediately following her postgraduate training, she was invited to join the Yale faculty. She became an active clinician, and director of the Department of Psychiatry's Adult Inpatient Acute-Treatment Program at Yale–New Haven Hospital, as well as an active researcher.

Dr. Mazure has been an invited speaker both nationally and internationally regarding her research on stress and depression, including presentations at the National Aeronautic and Space Administration and at the Smithsonian Institution, and she has been featured on ABC's *Primetime Live* and the BBC/Discovery Health documentary *The Science of Stress*. She was invited by Tipper Gore to participate in The First White House Conference on Mental Health; by Donna E. Shalala, the Secretary of Health and Human Services, to the Bi-National Israel–USA Conference entitled Promoting Women's Health Across Generations; and by the American Psychological Association to chair the Summit on Women and Depression at the Wye River Plantation.

In directing *Women's Health Research at Yale*, Dr. Mazure oversees an extensive research portfolio investigating sex and gender differences across many medical and behavioral content areas. These areas range from studies on cardiovascular health, depression, and osteoporosis to breast cancer, autoimmune disorders, and domestic violence. In addition, she leads a number of research and training initiatives focusing on the importance of gender in understanding behavioral health. She is the principal investigator for a number of programs at Yale funded by the National Institutes of Health (NIH), including the Yale Interdisciplinary Women's Health Research Scholar Program on Women and Drug Abuse, and the Sex-Specific Factors Core of the Transdisciplinary Tobacco Use Research Center studying sex-specific factors in nicotine dependence and treatment. She also is the scientific director of Yale's Specialized Center of Research on Women's Health: Sex, Stress, and Cocaine Addiction, which is also funded by NIH.

Translating research findings into policy has become an increasingly important goal for Dr. Mazure. She has provided invited testimony before Congress on several occasions regarding the importance of research on women's health. She has been the invited speaker on issues of pressing need in women's health at the Permanent Commission on the Status of Women for the State of Connecticut and at the United States Congressional Women's Caucus. She also has served as a public health fellow for the Committee on Government Reform of the U.S. House of Representatives.

Dr. Mazure has been the honored recipient of awards including a U.S. Public Health Service Fellowship and the Stephen Fleck Clinician and Teacher Award at Yale University School of Medicine. She is a fellow of the American Psychological Association and is on the editorial boards of the *Journal of Women's Health* and *Experimental and Clinical Psychopharmacology.*

Gwendolyn Puryear Keita, PhD, is the executive director of the Public Interest (PI) Directorate of the American Psychological Association (APA). Before assuming that position, she was director of the APA Women's Programs Office. She has coauthored several books and journal articles and presented extensively on women's issues, women's health in particular, and work, stress, and health. She has convened three conferences on psychosocial and behavioral factors in women's health and is coeditor of *Health Care and Women: Psychological, Social, and Behavioral Influences* (1997).

Dr. Keita is also coeditor of *Women and Depression: Risk Factors and Treatment Issues* (1990), the report on the APA Women and Depression Task Force. She also coauthored *No Safe Haven: Male Violence Against Women at Home, at Work, and in the Community* (1994), the Report of the APA Committee on Women in Psychology's Task Force on Male Violence Against Women. The report reviewed psychological research and made recommendations for interventions, legal changes, and policy initiatives. Dr. Keita convened the Summit on Women and Depression (2000), coedited a special edition of the *Journal of Affective Disorders* (2004), and special sections of the *Psychology of Women Quarterly* (2003) and *Professional Psychology: Research and Practice* (2003) on women and depression.

Dr. Keita was instrumental in developing the new field of occupational health psychology, has convened five international conferences on occupational stress and health, and coauthored several books and journal articles on the subject. These books include: *An Agenda for the 1990s* (1992); *Job Stress in a Changing Workforce: Investigating Gender, Diversity, and Family Issues* (1994); and *Job Stress Interventions* (1995). Dr. Keita has presented before Congress on depression, violence, and other issues.